Lectures on
The ART of Surgery

Lectures on
The ART of Surgery

Chief Editor

Harsha Jauhari

MS FRCS FICS FAIS FISOT Dip Medi Ethics & Law
Dr BC Roy National Awardee
Chairman
Department of Renal Transplant Surgery
Sir Ganga Ram Hospital
New Delhi, India

Co-Editor

Ashish Dey

MS FMAS FIAGES FACS
Senior Consultant
Department of Laparoscopic and General Surgery
Sir Ganga Ram Hospital
New Delhi, India

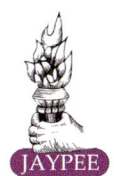

JAYPEE BROTHERS MEDICAL PUBLISHERS
The Health Sciences Publisher
New Delhi | London

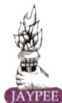 **Jaypee Brothers Medical Publishers (P) Ltd**

Headquarters
EMCA House
23/23-B, Ansari Road, Daryaganj
New Delhi 110 002, India
Landline: +91-11-23272143, +91-11-23272703
+91-11-23282021, +91-11-23245672
E-mail: jaypee@jaypeebrothers.com

Corporate Office
Jaypee Brothers Medical Publishers (P) Ltd.
4838/24, Ansari Road, Daryaganj
New Delhi 110 002, India
Phone: +91-11-43574357
Fax: +91-11-43574314
E-mail: jaypee@jaypeebrothers.com

Overseas Office
JP Medical Ltd.
83, Victoria Street, London
SW1H 0HW (UK)
Phone: +44-20 3170 8910
E-mail: info@jpmedpub.com

EU GPSR Authorised Representative
Logos Europe, 9 rue Nicolas Poussin
17000, La Rochelle, France
Phone: +33 (0) 6 67 93 73 78
E-mail: Contact@logoseurope.eu

Website: www.jaypeebrothers.com
Website: www.jaypeedigital.com

Lectures on the ART of Surgery

First Edition: 2023, Reprint: 2025

ISBN: 978-93-5465-905-8

Printed in India

Contributors

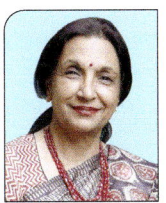

Abha Majumdar
Director and Head
Center of IVF and Human Reproduction
Sir Ganga Ram Hospital
New Delhi, India

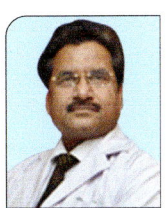

Ajay Sharma
Senior Consultant
Department of Urology
Sir Ganga Ram Hospital
New Delhi, India

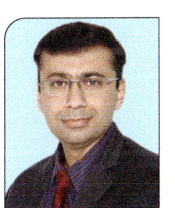

Ajay Yadav
Vice Chairman and Senior Consultant
Institute of Vascular and Endovascular Sciences
Sir Ganga Ram Hospital
New Delhi, India

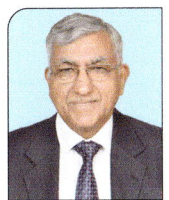

AK Grover
Chairman
Department of Ophthalmology
Sir Ganga Ram Hospital
New Delhi, India

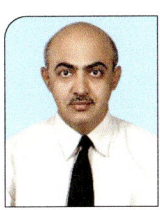

Anil Arora
Chairman and Director of GI Endoscopy
Department of Gastroenterology and Hepatology
Sir Ganga Ram Hospital
New Delhi, India

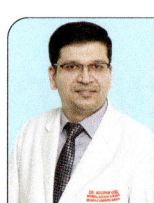
Anupam Goel
Consultant
Max Institute of Minimal Access
Bariatric and Robotic Surgery
Max Superspeciality Hospital,
Mohali, Punjab, India

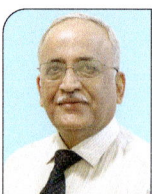
Anurag Krishna
Chairman
Pediatrics and Pediatric Surgery
Max Institute of Pediatrics
Max Healthcare Institute
New Delhi, India

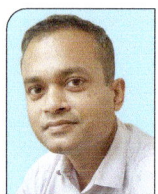
Ashish Dey MS FMAS FIAGES FACS
Senior Consultant
Department of Laparoscopic and General Surgery
Sir Ganga Ram Hospital
New Delhi, India

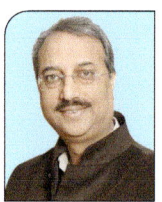
Chand Wattal
Chairman
Institute of Clinical Microbiology and Immunology
Sir Ganga Ram Hospital
New Delhi, India

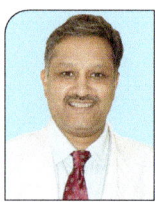
Deep Goel
Senior Director and Head
Department of Surgical Gastroentero Onco
Robotics and Advance Laparoscopy and Bariatric Surgery
BLK-MAX Superspeciality Hospital
New Delhi, India

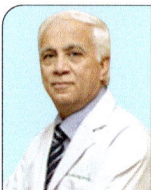
Devinder Rai
Senior Consultant
Department of ENT
Sir Ganga Ram Hospital
New Delhi, India

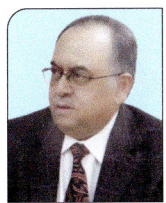

Harsha Jauhari
Chairman
Department of Renal Transplant Surgery
Sir Ganga Ram Hospital
New Delhi, India

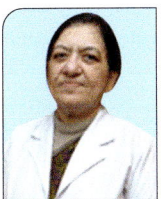

Harsha Khullar
Senior Consultant
Department of Obstetrics and Gynecology
Sir Ganga Ram Hospital
New Delhi, India

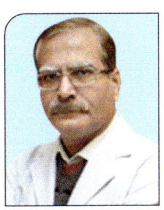

Ish Anand
Senior Consultant
Department of Neurology
Sir Ganga Ram Hospital
New Delhi, India

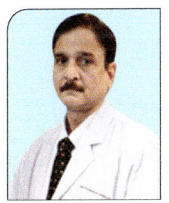

KK Saxena
Senior Consultant and Chairperson
Department of Radiology
Sir Ganga Ram Hospital
New Delhi, India

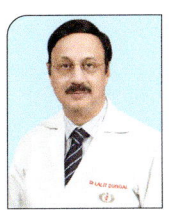

Lalit Duggal
Senior Consultant and Chairman
Department of Rheumatology and Clinical Immunology
Sir Ganga Ram Hospital
New Delhi, India

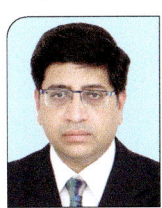

Naresh Dua
Senior Consultant
Department of Anesthesiology, Pain and Perioperative Medicine
Sir Ganga Ram Hospital
New Delhi, India

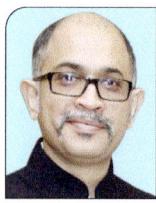

Niraj Tyagi
Consultant
Institute of Critical Care Medicine
Sir Ganga Ram Hospital
New Delhi, India

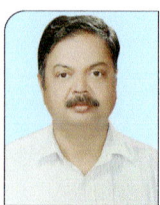

PK Agarwal
Senior Consultant
Department of Medicine
Sir Ganga Ram Hospital
New Delhi, India

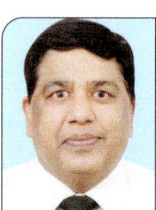

Pradeep Jain
Director–Pain Services
Vice-Chairperson
Institute of Anesthesiology, Pain and Perioperative Medicine
Sir Ganga Ram Hospital
New Delhi, India

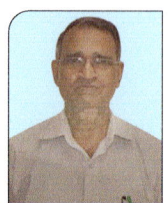

R Sarangi
Senior Consultant
Department of Laparoscopic, Laser and General Surgery
Sir Ganga Ram Hospital
New Delhi, India

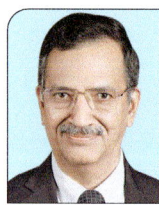

Rajesh Khullar
Senior Director
Institute of Laparoscopic
Endoscopic and Bariatric Surgery
Max Superspeciality Hospital
New Delhi, India

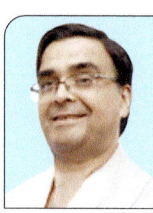

Rajiv Parekh
Chairman
Division of Peripheral Vascular and Endovascular Sciences
Medanta–The Medicity
Gurugram, Haryana, India

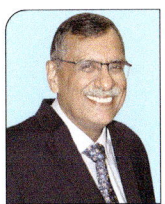

Rakesh Kumar Khazanchi
Chairman
Department of Plastic
Aesthetic and Reconstructive Surgery
Medanta–The Medicity
Gurugram, Haryana, India

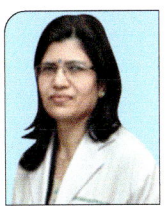

Rashmi Jain
Senior Consultant
Department of Anesthesiology, Pain and Perioperative Medicine
Sir Ganga Ram Hospital
New Delhi, India

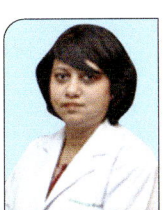

Sanghamitra Datta
Senior Consultant
Institute of Clinical Microbiology and Immunology
Sir Ganga Ram Hospital
New Delhi, India

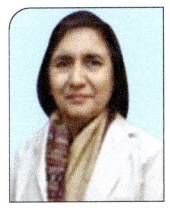

Sunita Bhalla
Senior Consultant
Department of Pathology
Sir Ganga Ram Hospital
New Delhi, India

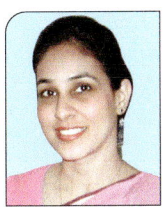

Vasundhara Oberoi
Senior Consultant
Department of Plastic and Cosmetic Surgery
Aesthetic Surgery Unit
Sir Ganga Ram Hospital
New Delhi, India

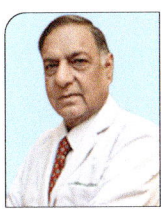

Vijay Arora
Senior Consultant
Department of Laparoscopy, Laser and General Surgery
Sir Ganga Ram Hospital
New Delhi, India

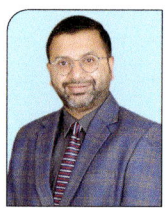

Vivek Bindal
Head of Department
Institute of Minimal Access, Bariatric and Robotic surgery
Max Superspeciality Hospitals
Noida, Uttar Pradesh, India

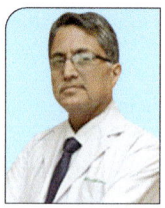

VK Nijhawan
Senior Consultant
Department of Orthopedics
Sir Ganga Ram Hospital
New Delhi, India

Message from the Editor's Desk

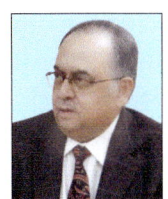

One of the great surgeons of our times, the late Dr KC Mahajan, in 2003, called me and said 'I am told that you are a good teacher, why don't you create a course for upcoming surgeons that will inspire them to become good, and safe surgeons?' I took this as a challenge and conceived a course on a facet of Surgery, which has been accepted as integral, but never given its due – The Art of Surgery.

The science of surgery is accepted, but the fact that it is performed in an "Operation Theater" is not emphasized.

Great surgeons make surgery look easy and boring. What they do or do not are equally important.

I asked senior surgeons to talk about various "Concepts and Attitudes", e.g., approach to a woman / child as a surgical patient or Pain–friend or foe.

Various younger consultants were asked to talk about how to perform Ward procedures. We had colleagues helping young trainee surgeons on the proper use of various "Surgical Tools". I requested various specialty Heads to discuss how they would approach a Polytrauma patient, as a first responder: Pregnant woman, turn left side or right side up?; multiple fractures: limb to be straightened or not? Baby injured – treat or scoop and scoot?

The combined experience and knowledge of almost 50 consultants, brought to bear on the "How" of surgery, has been one of the most enriching experiences of my life.

The doctors involved in this journey are indicated in the book. Over the years another great surgeon Dr Samiran Nundy, Dean of GRIPMER and its staff led by Mr Sansar Chand has given unstinted advice and support.

My thanks to Dr Rashmi Saluja, Executive Chairperson, Religare Enterprises Limited, a dear friend, for her unquestioning support in providing funds for the publishing of this book.

It is a leap of faith and an industry first for Care Health Insurance to support educational/ upskilling/training initiatives of medical professionals.

The publishers, Jaypee Brothers Medical Publishers (P) Ltd have been very supportive and accommodative. They have constantly tried to maintain the highest standards of publishing and have cooperated in last minute changes against a tight schedule.

The Chairman and Management of SGRH, led by my friend and an Eminent Nephrologist Dr DS Rana, has been totally positive and encouraging in this venture, giving unstinting support.

The Ethicon Foundation has also been involved over the years and provided practice JJGS and equipment for skill development. We look to taking this relationship forward in the years to come.

Over the years, The ASICON CME Foundation, through its convenor, Dr SB Agarwal and co-convenor Dr Vinod K Malik, has been funding various CME activities. I, as its President, have tried to bring in a new dimension, and business module, for Teachers/Students to publish Booklets/Magazines/Journals, under its aegis.

Dr Ashish Dey, my co-editor has been a revelation over the past few years. He has taken over the entire responsibility of compiling / editing/ corresponding etc. of this project. He is the epitome of what a young talented, aspiring surgeon should be.

Finally, my wife, Dr Seema, who has long ago stopped trying to figure out what goes on in my mind, but gives me immense strength, advice, and has taught me "everything that you know"!!

My thanks to my surgical gurus, colleagues and friends who have, over the years, provided unswerving and unquestioned encouragement.

If this book can help generate and demonstrate the beauty of an operation, in the hands of a young surgeon, it will have fulfilled its purpose.

Harsha Jauhari
MS FRCS FICS FAIS FISOT Dip Medi Ethics & Law
Dr BC Roy National Awardee
Chairman
Department of Renal Transplant Surgery
Sir Ganga Ram Hospital and Artemis Health Institute
Gurugram, Haryana, India

Message from the Co-Editor's Desk

The book "Lectures on the ART of Surgery" marks the culmination of the efforts of two decades of intensive teaching classes, in Sir Ganga Ram Hospital, by the pioneers of their respective departments. As a co-editor, I owe all the authors and contributors to the book a debt of gratitude for their efforts. As I follow Dr Jauhari's footsteps, I also understand the efforts that took him to firstly organize the classes for so many years, do the transcription from spoken lectures and finally collating into the book.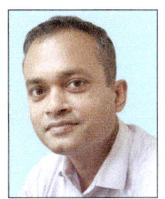

With this, we also do acknowledge that the field of surgery undergoes phenomenal changes every year and cannot all be covered in a book. This is not a textbook in the true sense and does not cover the entire gamut of the particular topic dealt here. This book, as the name suggests, dwells on the "Art" rather than the science of surgery that is outlined in the first part of the book. This is the "penumbra" of the surgical skills, that every upcoming young surgeon needs to know and inculcate within himself. The other three parts includes surgical acumen in wards, roadside trauma and surgical "tools".

As the first surgeon co-editor of the book, I believe many more steps need to be planned and implemented toward the future of surgical training for Residents and young surgeons. The book is a first small step toward that direction.

Ashish Dey
MS FMAS FIAGES FACS
Senior Consultant
Department of Laparoscopic and General Surgery
Sir Ganga Ram Hospital
New Delhi, India

Foreword

"Lectures on the ART of Surgery" is a collection of the last 2 decades of teachings in the "ART of Surgery" classes organized in Sir Ganga Ram Hospital which cover the essential knowledge required for a safe surgery. This book prepares the trainees and the trained surgeons alike to enable them to come out victorious in the battleground of the operation theater.

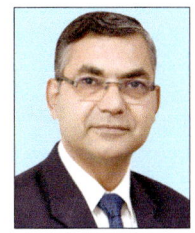

The book is an easy reading and covers topics which are otherwise not easily available in textbooks and I would like to recommend it as must read to all trainee surgeons.

Pawanindra Lal
MS DNB FIMSA FCLS FRCS FRCSEd
FRCSGlasg FRCSEng FACS FAMS
Director-Professor of Surgery
Maulana Azad Medical College
Executive Director and CEO
National Board of Examinations in Medical Sciences

Foreword

It is well-accepted aphorism that surgery is both "a science" and "an art". While the "science" of surgery is deliberated upon regularly both in textbooks, journals, and conferences, it is the "art" of surgery that gets a short shrift. The practice of this "art" gets fillip through this book.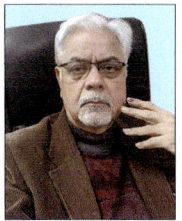

The comprehensive management of patients, surgical or otherwise requires knowledge, skills, attitude, communication, professionalism, and problem solving. While there are many sources to acquire knowledge, there are but fewer such resources addressing the other domains.

This book is majorly focused on how to apply knowledge to improve the outcome and experience of surgical patients.

Another important aspect that this book addresses, is how to be an efficient young surgeon in control of a situation that can be at times very demanding and challenging. As they say "anger management makes one calm person", for surgeons the equivalent of that is to avoid panic. Panic makes for poor decisions and poorer outcomes, yet it is part of one's DNA; can one avoid altogether? One way is to be aware of possible scenarios and be mentally prepared to manage such situations. This book deals with this aspect in a very effective way.

Though the subjects chosen are across the large spectrum of surgical specialties, however, the theme is basic and targets new entrants. This is about what a first responder, new to his trade, will like to possess, to navigate his way around; be it a casualty call, assisting in "Operation Room" or looking after the patient in postoperative situation. The wisdom of well-chosen specialists in the field will definitely come in handy.

I have no doubt that this labor of love of Dr Harsha Jauhari will prove to be the modern day version of the venerable Pye's Surgical Handicraft of the years gone by.

Vinod K Malik MS
Chairman
Department of Laparoscopic and General Surgery
Dean, GRIPMER
Sir Ganga Ram Hospital
New Delhi, India

Foreword

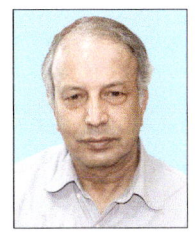

If there ever was a time such a book was sorely needed it is now. The so-called up-to-date and modern surgeons have become so immersed in technology for diagnosis and treatment with CT scans, PET CTs, MRIs and Angiograms that most of them have forgotten the art of talking to a patient and explaining what they think is wrong. They spend their time trying to convince them that a costly robotic procedure is what they badly need when there are many simpler alternatives.

I think reading and rereading this book will bring us all down to earth. We will be reminded that when we deal with human beings, we have to begin by talking to them kindly and touching them. Taking a good history and performing a careful clinical examination is now a dying art, but it is much more valuable and necessary than all the so called "science" that is constantly being thrown at us.

I therefore welcome this important publication and am honored to have been asked to write a message.

Samiran Nundy
MA MChir FRCS FRCP
Advisor
Department of Surgical Gastroenterology and
Liver Transplantation
Sir Ganga Ram Hospital
New Delhi, India

Acknowledgments

We wish to acknowledge the help of all the authors for their valuable time, especially because they met the tight deadline set by us, by working fast and still make outstanding contributions, to make it possible to bring out this book. The students and enthusiasts who love the field of critical care medicine who are always avidly waiting for something new to read, most of all deserve our thanks.

Our thanks are due to our students who inspire us to teach and colleagues who allow us to do the work peacefully and our families who tolerate our inaccessibility while we are working to bring out this book.

We are especially thankful to Ms Chetna Malhotra (Senior Director – Professional Publishing, Marketing and Business Development), and Ms Saima Rashid (Manager Publishing) of M/s Jaypee Brothers Medical Publishers (P) Ltd, New Delhi, India, for giving a go-ahead at the very beginning and helping us in every way possible to bring out this book.

Last but not the least, our prayers and thanks to the Almighty for blessing us in this task.

Contents

SECTION 2: Surgeon and His Tools

SECTION 3: Young Surgeon as the First Responder

SECTION 4: Ward Procedure Skills

Introduction

How do some surgeons make operations look boring and unexciting? "Big deal... Even I can do this" ... is the reaction they evoke in onlookers. This is surgery at its best.. the surgeon has removed almost all the possible pitfalls and is performing without any strain. Why are some surgeons "hemorrhagic".... they touch anything it bleeds ? While there are some others who are "hemostatic"; they are summoned to help, they just touch the patient and the bleeding stops!

Again, some surgeons put in a finger and pull out the appendix 10 times out of 10, while others pull out everything but the appendix!

Some clinicians are called in the middle of the night, when everyone else has tried and failed, and put in a Ryles tube, or Urinary catheter or I.V. drip in the first attempt.

Some nurses, clinicians can give painless intramuscular, intravenous injections or lumber punctures, while others are not so painless!! Some can just readjust your pillow or position and provide untold comfort.

There are countless other examples of the "How" coming into play when the "What", "When" and "Why" are being undertaken. It is this "How" that is the understated "Art of Surgery" which differentiates the great and good practitioner from the average. He or she may not even be aware of what they are doing differently, but they are making that difference - we need to find out what it is. All Surgeons follow the science, the techniques, the procedures - but in some hands it is poetry in motion.

It is calculated that in any operation, in one hour of surgery, only 17 minutes are repetitive and wasted better than average surgeons, do away with the 43 minutes of fuss, stretch the 17 minutes into 30 minutes of slow, comfortable movements. They look like they are wasting time and yet finish, successfully, well before others.

Unnecessary drama means, neither the surgeon nor anyone else knows what is going on. Do it once, Do it well!!

This book is an attempt to compile and present the experience of a large number of very senior, senior and young colleagues, across a wide spectrum of specialties, to glean from them the hidden gems of knowledge that they take for granted. It is said that in the formative years of a surgeon, he is exposed to around 20 surgical teachers, and they have been exposed to 20 teachers as well. So, in one generation, a young surgeon gets the benefit of almost 400 surgeons. That is why an average surgeon is a very good surgeon, having success in the 90-plus percents. A great surgeon has a success rate in the mid 90%'s. A once in a generation surgeon has success rates in the 97-98%'s. The gap between an average and an outstanding surgeon is those few vital percents!!

More & more procedures are getting "modernized" into hi-tech exercise. The hands- on approach of the conventional and to some extent, endoscopic procedures are being overtaken by laparoscopic and now robotic technology. And yet, good basic surgical skills, inculcated at the young surgeons training phase, will always hold its own at crucial times, a good surgeon will always be a good surgeon, no matter what the armamentaria being used is.

Some of the Lectures were amenable to transcription, but some parts of them were demonstrative and therefore, difficult to put down on paper. Any shortfall or deficit is necessarily to be attributed to the editors.

Should this book evoke artistic sparks in some young surgeons, our vision shall be fulfilled.

After all, surgery is conducted not in an Operation Laboratory, but in an Operation Theater!

Harsha Jauhari

Concepts and Attitude

Surgical Deportment and Opinion: I Think, Therefore I am

Harsha Jauhari

■ INTRODUCTION

Surgical deportment and surgical opinion defines a surgeon. The ABC of successful surgical practice and temperament may be spelt out as Availability, Behavior, and Competence, in that order. There is no point in being extremely competent, but never available to a patient who needs you. The "A" of ABC also stands for appearance, which is very important. You cannot improve your looks, but what you can do is to try to present yourself in the best possible manner. You should be well groomed, with a decent haircut, and should be clean shaven or have a well-trimmed beard or moustache. Your clothes need not be new, but should be clean and pressed. Your shoes should not be dirty. Generally, the same rules apply to women surgeons. You should avoid slouching and should not look sloppy. These details play a part in defining your temperament.

■ APPEARANCE

As far as appearance is concerned, the importance of a uniform can never be underestimated. Consider that while soldiers, surgeons, chefs, and criminals all use the knife, only the first three wear a uniform at work. The uniform indicates that they are bound by certain rules, a common code of conduct. People are also more likely to have greater confidence in those who wear uniforms. Even when soldiers, surgeons, and chefs are not in uniform, most of them tend to behave in a fashion consistent with their profession. Criminals use their weapon indiscriminately, but surgeons, soldiers and chefs use their knife professionally. A criminal is answerable to nobody and, therefore, follows no rules. He inspires no confidence. So, the importance of a uniform can never be underestimated.

■ BEHAVIOR

Your behavior is a reflection of your outlook toward and empathy for the patient, and defines your temperament in the context of surgery and life in general. Temperament is important and self-explanatory. Unlike physicians (to some extent), philosophers and artists, a surgeon cannot afford to be eccentric. Further, you should not only have a good knowledge of your field, but should also be able to inspire confidence through your behavior. Philosophers, painters, and pianists by tradition are eccentric. It is not for surgeons. Surgeons are not eccentric or not expected to be eccentric. Behavior is also important. The patient who walks in is worried and has to be reassured. He is ignorant and, therefore, scared. He will be going into unknown territory, where he will be sleeping. Things are going to happen to him when he is unconscious and then he will have to be brought back safely from his sleep. You need to explain the matter to him so that he feels confident that he is in safe hands. He is supposed to go to a territory which is unknown where he is going to be sleeping. Things are going to happen to his unconscious body and then also has to be brought back safely from his sleep.

Therefore, it is unacceptable to behave rudely with your patients. Patients or their attendants occasionally act rude, but you have to take it in your stride and be nice to them, so long as your self-respect remains intact. Rudeness on the part of the paramedical staff can be excused occasionally, but you cannot afford to be rude. If you are labeled as an ill-tempered and badly behaved person, your colleagues will no longer be willing to help you. Also, you should never bad-mouth a colleague or damage his reputation. Frowning at another surgeon's prescription or making sarcastic comments is completely unacceptable because what goes around comes around. Most doctors try to give their best. Besides, patients never think well of a doctor who speaks ill of another doctor. You may not have the same opinion as the other doctor, which is completely fine.

The approach you adopt toward your patients should be consistent with your temperament. If you like being friendly, your patients will be happy that you are friendly. Whatever is in keeping with your temperament—whether it is being friendly, remote, mature, or grave—you should develop it and make it a part of your professional attitude. One might get to be known as a person who is sober or as a jolly person or as a friendly person but committed and serious. Also to be noted that life will not always be nice to you. There will be good days and bad days, both on the personal and professional fronts. If you have an image that is second nature to you, you can retreat into it and still be able to meet the demands of your profession, keeping that image intact on the outside.

■ CONFIDENCE

Confidence is very important and should go hand in hand with competence. Many surgeons are confident, but very laid back. Unless somebody pushes them to do something, they do not do it and if they do, they are not likely to do it very well. On the other hand, many surgeons are more confident than competent, which is a dangerous thing. At some point in his career, every surgeon feels that he is experienced enough to handle virtually any problem that comes his way. This is the stage which is the most dangerous. Surgery is a great leveler. Days can be unpredictably difficult and long. Overconfidence blinds the sensible and reasoning mind. Confidence comes with knowledge and talent is honed by experience. A lot of hard work is required to build these up. The surgeon has to work harder on the areas in which he is relatively weak and he will surely improve. When the surgeon is assessing the patient in the outpatient clinic, the patient or attendant, too, are forming their opinion of him. They are in the process of determining whether he can be trusted, whether he has the expertise that he claims to have and whether he appears confident enough to handle any complications that may crop up. A patient takes roughly 30 seconds to decide whether he wants a surgery to be performed by a particular surgeon. One has to try to be that surgeon.

Not all of us are born to be world-class champions like Schumacher. Most of us are born with limited talent, but we can all become good drivers. All said and done, an average surgeon is a very good surgeon. Dexterity can mostly be imbibed. Considering everything, the outcome of surgery depends on how well you perform on the table. What is important is to perform the operation perfectly.

Join the Race or be Left Behind—"Staying Abreast"

Harsha Jauhari

■ INTRODUCTION

The topic "joining the race" is inappropriate because "all surgeons are leaders". Always. There is no democracy when it comes to the operating table. The surgeon is the only leader. One cannot operate by consensus. The surgeon is the team leader and takes the decisions; the other people are there only to assist him. This is unmistakable. A surgeon grows in his profession through his capacity to make decisions and provide leadership. He graduates from being the leader of the unit to being the best known surgeon in the hospital and subsequently, the best known in his specialty, and his sphere of influence expands as he goes along. The notion of any surgeon being "left behind" is unthinkable and unacceptable. No surgeon will ever be left behind, and should not be left behind.

It is important to understand the attributes of a surgeon as a leader. All leaders strive for excellence. An average surgeon is a very good surgeon. He has outcome rates of >90%. An outcome rate of 50% would mean that half the patients would die and half would get better, which is unacceptable. An outstanding surgeon has a success rate of 96–97% and an absolutely brilliant surgeon probably has a success rate of 97–98% or 99%, but nobody will ever have 100% success. There is very little difference between the success rates of an average surgeon and an absolutely brilliant surgeon, and though those few percentage points matter, good surgeons should never be negative or defensive about their outcomes because they are constantly striving for excellence.

Surgeons have to be able to make decisions—hard decisions, and sometimes, cruel decisions. Your excellence or experience comes into play during surgical decision-making. To an extent, surgeons tend to be dogmatic because there is no room for considerations like "Do we?", "Do we not?", "Shall we?", and "Shall we not?". A surgical decision cannot be graded; you cannot operate by percentages. Either you perform an operation or you do not. When you decide, it is either a 100% "Yes" or an absolute "No". You neither see the grades, nor do you want to see them. You cannot perform a 70% laparotomy because somebody has said he is 70% sure. You either do it or you do not. Then, of course, you should be able to see your decision through. If you believe that you are doing the right thing on the basis of good facts and see it through, then you must accept the responsibility for the outcome. He should have shoulders broad enough to accept the responsibility for the outcomes.

Decision-making requires experience and a thorough knowledge of the standard procedures. You cannot escape the fact that you need to put in hard work and gain a basic knowledge of procedures. However, to become a leader and move ahead, you have to acquire a wide and profound knowledge of the recent and current developments in other parts of the world. Textbooks are not the ideal source of current guidelines and evidence. The material in most recent editions of a book is based on statistics and facts that were relevant a good decade earlier. As it takes almost 2 years to bring out textbooks, they are already outdated by the time they are published. In today's world, it is necessary to keep oneself up to date through journals, conferences, and the internet.

Personal experience, insight, and intuition are also very important. You can gain experience only with time. The experience of colleagues and sometimes, an intuition that what you are doing is right, also matter. You may not always know the reasons, which might become clear to you later. But you should still go ahead and do what you believe is right.

It is important to "seize the moment". One has to keep in touch with new innovations and new techniques. Endoscopic and laparoscopic techniques had ushered in a revolution in the 1990s. They brought about a sea change in the way a few surgeries or procedures were performed. Then came robotic surgeries, which have become the standard of care in the case of many diseases. Laparoscopy could be well-suited for renal transplantation and might be the next revolution in transplant surgery. When laparoscopy arrived on the scene, many surgeons realized that it was here to stay. They seized on the technique when it came. "Adapt, adopt, and project" is the way ahead because once you have perfected it; you will be one of the few people who knows what he is talking about. Then, of course, you have to project yourself. In the beginning, you have to do a bit of self-advertisement. The press, television, and various conferences are the media through which you can project your expertise.

All surgeons contribute to progress in their lifetime, in one way or the other. There are three types of progress. There is one type in which surgeons find a better way of doing something—a new way, new technique, or new approach. For example, in the middle of the last century, various gastrectomies were performed to excise peptic ulcers. Then came vagotomies followed by highly selective vagotomies. Surgeons tried to improve upon surgeries and innovated to come up with superior surgical techniques and modifications to the procedure. The results improved. You can do the same thing in a simpler, cheaper, less morbid, and less time-consuming manner to obtain better results. Performing the same surgery, but with less effort can also be considered progress.

Using a new technique that makes previous procedures obsolete is progress. Laparoscopic techniques for gallbladder calculi and endoscopic techniques for renal and ureteric calculi led to a huge reduction in morbidity and greatly improved the outcomes of surgeries. Open cholecystectomy and pyelolithotomies were awful operations, no matter how well they were performed, and involved a large, painful incision. Subcostal incisions for cholecystectomy or the flank incisions for nephrolithotomy or ureterolithotomy were associated with terribly high morbidity. Endoscopic techniques make these procedures virtually painless and the vast majority of patients are discharged without major problems. The size of the stone to be taken out determines the size of the incision for access. Thus, the same operation becomes simpler, is associated with lower morbidity, involves less time and fewer antibiotics, and has good results. That is progress in the real sense.

Now for the third type of progress, with the arrival of cimetidine, the whole field of peptic ulcer surgery was wiped out. A generation ago, the yardstick of a good surgeon was how quickly he could perform a partial gastrectomy. Now, gastrectomy is seldom found in the main operation theater (OT) list of hospitals. Because of proton pump inhibitors, vagotomies and gastrectomies are no longer performed for peptic ulcers. Also, emergency surgeries for bleeding or perforation are rare. That, I believe, is also progress.

Panic and the Surgeon: "To Fuse or Defuse"

Harsha Jauhari

■ INTRODUCTION

"If you can keep your head when all about you are losing theirs and blaming it on you, If you can trust yourself when all men doubt you, but make allowance for their doubting too!" said the famous Rudyard Kipling, exhorting us to maintain our self-confidence in times of doubt. Jean Kerr, on the other hand, said, "If you can keep your head when all about you are losing theirs, it is just possible that you have not grasped the situation." In this case, you are completely oblivious to the repercussions of the situation and are being totally indifferent or you may be, as in the former situation, keeping calm and trying to defuse the crisis in a composed and methodical manner, which is what makes a surgeon.

Sudden, stressful situations give rise to an adrenergic response of fright and flight or fight. The "flight or fight" response is ingrained in the psyche of most four-legged animals in the wild. In the operating room, however, "flight" is not possible. Fright, therefore, has to be understood and tamed and converted to a useful "fight" response. How you go about this makes or breaks you as a surgeon and proves if you have "it" in you. It is not easy to develop nerves of steel and you can do so only after you have seen others handling such trying situations efficiently and tactfully. It is, of course, human to be afraid and panic. Ultimately, all surgeons are human. How you overcome your fear determines your caliber and stature as a surgeon in the future.

From our basic surgical training and the fables passed down the corridors of medicine, we have learnt that hemorrhage occurs often enough, but it is very rare for a patient to lose his life because of it. This means that the methods employed are usually successful. It also means that we can understand, analyze, and employ these methods when required. There is a way out of potentially difficult situations. The trick is to make these methods efficient and reproducible.

You may face panic in three situations: (1) the patient or his attendants are in panic, (2) a colleague is in panic and seeks your assistance, and (3) you are in panic.

1. In the first instance, you are not panicking and you have to try to understand why the patient or his attendants are panicking. Is it that the patient has suddenly collapsed because he has been told he requires surgery, or does he fear malignancy, or is his panic due to economic reasons? A few patients panic due to the economic repercussions of a disabling, debilitating, or devastating disease. If reassurance is required, it is important to "educate" the patient and his relatives, address the root cause and reassure them. If intervention is required, you have to intervene.

2. In the second situation, your colleague is in panic, but you are not. The situation can go two ways—either you also start to panic or you try to control the panic. It is important to assess the problem and decide if it is for you to bring the situation under control. If not, then decide whose assistance should be sought. Do not leave the operation room. Give whatever support you can till suitable help arrives. If it is you who are at the helm, you must remain composed, summon help, gather all resources, think laterally and assess as many options as possible. Then proceed. You may need to ask the original operating surgeon to "sit down" and take a break, but do it gracefully. For example, you might say, "please go and have a cup of coffee or tea. We will call you when necessary." You should be decorous because one day, you might be in the other person's shoes.

3. There are many situations which may cause you to panic. These include hemorrhage on the table, the operation not going as planned, friable bowel, vitreous prolapse and meningocele rupture. Similarly, a cardiac or anesthetic event may lead to panic, as may be a surgical misadventure. It is said that "the swiftest way an unconscious patient retaliates to an incompetent surgeon is by hemorrhage". The best way of tackling a hemorrhage is by preventing it, anticipating it and knowing the techniques required to control it.

Panic control: Clamp down on all emotions. Do not shout, blame others, or repeat orders. Take charge and let the people around you know that you are going to lead the way and slow down. This is a paradox where you will actually be more effective if you appear to be in control. Make clean, deliberate, and purposeful movements. Absorb the panic of the others. If you are religious, mentally chant whatever "mantra" appeals to you and keep repeating it while you are managing the situation. It works! Mantras have an innate rhythm and chanting them imbues one's breathing with a rhythm that helps to control one's mind.

Surgery is not for the faint-hearted. You need to have nerves of steel to deal with the kinds of situations you will inevitably face in your lifetime. It is but natural to be afraid. "Only a block of wood does not experience panic." Panic is created by an adrenergic response to a situation. In this state, people can flee or fight in response to extraordinary pain. That is using the situation to your advantage, rather than reducing yourself to a "quivering jellyfish". Therefore, "panic controlled is controlled panic". And "controlled panic is battle won!" I conclude with two relevant quotes:

> "Fire is the test of gold; adversity, of strong men"
>
> —*Seneca*

> "A wounded deer leaps highest"
>
> —*Emily Dickinson*

Self-doubt, Self-audit, Self-reliance—Optimizing Competence: Confidence Ratio

Harsha Jauhari

■ INTRODUCTION

This is a subject which is more philosophical than surgical, but it is important for every surgeon to have this in the mind. Self-doubt is important, and even more so for a surgeon. You must have doubt in yourself. It helps you to excel in your field. Self-audit is something you do yourself very intensely personal; it is not done in a group. Nobody can fool you except yourself, so if you are doing something, you must be very honest with yourself. "Am I doing this right, am I good enough, am I prepared?" However, too much of self-doubt can turn you into a nervous wreck, making you are incapable of doing anything. So, it has to be a contained, controlled type of doubt. Never let it become uncontrolled. Moderate doubt will lead you to wisdom.

Self-doubt may take many forms. When you are about to do something, you may be assailed by questions such as: "Can I do it? Am I good enough? Do I know enough? What happens if I fail? What will others say?" These are the thoughts that come to everyone of our mind. "Am I exposing myself, my ignorance in front of other people?" Suppose you are attending a conference where somebody is talking some rubbish and you know that he is talking rubbish, but you do not have the courage to challenge him. "What will people say?" Or you really do not understand what the person is saying, but you do not have the courage to stand up and ask, "I am sorry, I did not follow that" because you doubt yourself. Do not be afraid to doubt yourself.

There is nothing wrong with self-doubt. However, remember that nobody is perfect and that doubt is the first step toward truth. When you doubt something, you test what you are doubting and then come up with some ideas which lead you toward what is probably more correct. So, there is nothing wrong with self-doubt. As surgeons, you must all have it. If we did not have self-doubt, we would be like blocks of wood! To quote Amitabh Bachchan, "If I am happy and contended with my acting, I would stop growing. I need to be ignorant and hungry to be a better actor."

But having doubt in yourself is not enough. You have to take the next step, which is called self-audit. You have to take yourself to task in a very critical manner. Scan whatever you are doing. I feel everybody should audit their own cases. I may feel, I have done X number of cases of a particular disease. Relying on medical records is not a good idea. Making your own audit is important. What you felt, what you thought, what you recorded, how much was correct, how much was wrong,... it is very important to note down all this. It would be helpful for your publications, too. Start today. When you go home, make a note of what you did today. Write the salient features of each case. Periodically evaluate your perceptions of your knowledge.

When I was very young, my teacher told me, "there is no surgical examination which you can fail as long as you know Bailey and Love." This still holds true. A simple book like "Short Practice" and he never had the courage to call himself a textbook. That book contains virtually every bit of information the world needs today. You can expand on it, you can consult other books. As a super specialist, you can even dispute what the author wrote, but you cannot deny that what the book says is generally correct and generally safe and accepted in practice. No matter how well you know that book, you will always find something new which will surprise you. So test your knowledge and your perceptions of your knowledge. You think you know something. Go back to the book and read it. You may find something new. Keep testing and evaluating yourself.

A surgeon is always judged by his peers. It is good to pay heed to what your peers have to say. But at some point, you have to work differently from the others. The foundations may be the same, but you have to stand on your feet. You must also evaluate your judgments, which is where your records come in handy. "Why was I wrong repeatedly? Why am I right? If I am right, good. If I am wrong, why?" Compare your performance with that of your peers. Observe how other people operate. See whether you are doing it better, see whether you doing it worse. If they are doing something well, try to pick it up. Compare yourself with your seniors. Your seniors are not necessarily better. Be brutally honest, are you better than them? If yes, wonderful. If you are not as good as them, then learn.

Analyze your strengths. Whether you are a very good physician, or a very good technical surgeon, whatever it is, reinforce your skills. If you have certain weaknesses, be aware of them. For example, "I can never understand ECGs, I just cannot. If I can see an MI there, the patient is probably lying down in chest pain, either you accept your weakness as something which is not important in your field and get somebody else to do it, or keep trying to correct yourself. Cross-check discreetly. Analyze the impressions you receive from others. You may think you are wonderful, your colleagues may think you are not. You may think you are useless, while they may think that you are very good. So, discreetly cross check, you get the impressions. You never make a bit sure and be receptive to criticism in your work. Not all criticism is aimed at making you feel small. There are a lot of people who will offer genuine and positive criticism.

From self-audit, you must move to self-reliance. Always make sure that you are right and then go ahead. Self-reliance does not depend on anyone but yourself. If you want the job done well, do it yourself. Nobody will do it as well as you think it needs to be done.

A realistic self-assessment accompanied by inputs from your colleagues is the best foundation on which to build self-reliance. Listen to your friends, listen to your peers, and listen to your seniors. Remember that you are usually better than you think you are. A doctor is in the top 1% of the intelligence bracket. A person who has a postgraduate degree is in the top 0.1%. If you go beyond that, you are among the top 0.01%. So, you are much more intelligent than you think you are. You are not so stupid as you think you are and do not keep pulling yourselves down. We people are in the habit of pulling others down because we do not compare ourselves with people who have been in the same line of work for 10, 20, or 30 years or more than us. When you get to that stage, you may be as good or better than them, but you cannot grow before your time. Do not feel negative, think positively. Do not be afraid to stretch your abilities. If you are content with what you have, you will never progress. You will never progress. You have to stretch your abilities a little bit more anytime. Have you ever tried to lift a small cow? You will never be able to do it. But there are people who can lift a small cow because they have been lifting that cow since it was a calf. As the calf grew, their strength grew, so they are able to lift the cow. That is the way to grow stronger gradually with time. They can do what you cannot because they think they can. You have to think that you can do it, only then you will be able to do it. But if you give up in advance, you never will. You have to believe that there is nobody in the world who is better than you when you are doing a job. God above and me below, that is it. At the back of your mind, you may feel a lot of other things; but while you are doing something, the thought in the foreground must always be that you are the best, and then you will do it.

Now, this example perfectly conveys exactly what I am trying to say. If you want a thing done well, do it yourself. If you do not believe that you can do it yourself and always ask for help, you will probably never be able to do it. On the other hand, if you believe you can do it, but you do not have the required competence, you can get yourself into a mess. Now, the competence–confidence ratio is something very important. Your competence and your confidence must grow simultaneously. We do not want over competent surgeons who are underconfident; nor do we want overconfident people blundering around without competence. By and large, the ratio of competence and confidence should be 1. In other words, they should be matched. However, self-confidence is of utmost importance. As I have said very often, a surgeon should not be a follower. At the operating table, there is no democracy. You are the one and only surgeon. So, you have to lead and that requires self-confidence.

Competence is not static. You may be competent today, but you may be incompetent tomorrow. Keep in mind what the world is doing or you may be left behind. Confidence is not static either. You may be very confident at one point and you may not be confident at another. With certain operations, you feel very confident. With others, you may not be quite so confident. The stage of development also matters. From a student, you become a senior, then more senior, and then you become very senior. But with age, your agility starts declining. You have to accept that. It is a natural curve. Your confidence grows with experience, but then a stage comes when it starts going down. At every stage, you must self-audit. Keep rechecking, take help whenever required and be honest with yourself.

As surgeons we have to perform. We cannot theorize. I wonder if you have heard of General George Patton, one of the most famous surgeons general during World War II. He said "Take calculated risks but do not gamble. Let us try it, if he survives." We take calculated risks as surgeons. Physicians can theorize, surgeons have to perform and that is what is different from being rash. When you are aware of the risk, evaluate it and the chance of its working. Do it if you believe it will work. Whatever it is, do not be rash, never.

5

Conceptualization and Visualization of an Operation: Preparation for Surgery

Harsha Jauhari

■ INTRODUCTION

The physical problems that affect patients are similar. A hernia or a cataract or fibroid or a thyroid nodule will vary only in shape, size, or extent. What may differ is the approach to surgery when a combination of such problems occurs? An example is a pregnant woman with uterine fibroids, or associated cholecystitis, and hernia. A patient could have cardiac disease with renal failure. One can have diabetes coexisting with or causing cataract or a primary malignancy associated with pleural or pericardial effusions. Further, there may be some rare problems, such as purpura, jaundice, hemophilia, severe anemia, pulmonary edema, and malignant hypertension, in addition to the surgical problem.

Clearly, the approach to surgery cannot be the same in all the situations mentioned above. You have to gather all the relevant information well in advance, except in an emergency, because you cannot do so when you are at the table. You have to do it well in advance, except in an emergency. You have to think in your mind, which order they have to be addressed. For example, if you have to operate on a hernia and perform a cholecystectomy simultaneously, you will have to decide which one you should do first. There may be a reason why you want to perform the cholecystectomy first or why you want to do the hernia first. In a pregnant patient with uterine fibroids, you may want to get the baby out before dealing with the fibroids. You need to prioritize what you are going to do.

In a case of symptomatic cholecystitis with a coexisting small hernia, you may decide to tackle the simple hernia before dealing with the gallbladder. You might suddenly find that you have opened up a sliding hernia and the procedure has taken up the better part of the morning; the patient then unexpectedly develops an acute myocardial infarction and you have to abort the rest of the operation or it may happen that you open up a patient's abdomen, thinking he has acute appendicitis, but what you find is a tumor sitting over the cecum, which you have misdiagnosed and you have to perform a right hemicolectomy. Similarly, you might be planning to perform a straightforward gynecological surgery, but the operation suddenly turns life-threatening due to intraoperative bleeding and becomes a salvage operation. So, what you thought was simple turned out to be difficult. The operation has suddenly changed direction. What you were planning to do and what you end up doing may turn out to be totally different. You need to have backup plans for such exigencies. You have to consider in advance what might go wrong. You have to think of questions such as: "where could I go wrong and what would I do if something went wrong?"; "Have I involved the cardiologist beforehand?

Does he know this is a high-risk patient?"; "Is the anesthetist aware that there is a problem?"; and "Have I arranged for blood?"

In addition, try to be cognizant of situations which may arise months or years later because of what you have or have not done in your surgery. For example, you tie up the internal iliac arteries in a case of placenta previa with massive bleeding. Would this cause the patient problems later on? You might be tying up the carotid on one side due to trauma, without being aware that the other carotid is already blocked. Similarly, you may need to do extensive bowel resection for a patient, but you should be aware that in the years to come, he is going to suffer from malabsorption. Supposing you get many patients with ureteric calculi or renal calculi and in a very random, cavalier fashion, you opt for surgery, whether endoscopic or open. But you have not understood that every time you manipulate a ureter or the pelvis of the kidney, you are causing damage, which is going to heal by scarring. Thus, you have removed a stone, but the tendency to form stones remains. Another stone will be formed and this time, you have caused it. You have thus made the patient dependent on repeated surgery because of something you have done. So, try to take cognizance of these things when you are doing something. It is not enough to just operate and forget about it. Today, you might make a nice big incision for surgery for chronic renal failure and tomorrow, you might find that the patient needs a renal transplant and there is not enough space to make an incision for putting in a kidney. Such aspects have to be taken into account. The abdomen is not a playground or battleground for a multitude of incisions. Incisions have to be well thought out beforehand. Planning for any surgery is, therefore, crucial.

Straightforward problems have already been addressed by earlier generations of surgeons. For acute appendicitis, you perform an appendicectomy. Hernia repair is required for a hernia. For symptomatic gallbladder disease, you perform a cholecystectomy. All these are well-established procedures. You need to have a knowledge of the anatomy and the procedure concerned with all its variations. Combinations of problems may require more than one team. For example, you may be a gynecologist and the patient may have a preexisting problem for which you need to have a urologist or cardiac surgeon on standby, in case of emergency or you may need to inform the chest physician or blood bank before surgery. So, everybody has to be involved and other specialists must be told in advance so that they can plan accordingly. Your motto should be discuss and involve everyone; do not shy away from asking for help. Nobody ever thinks less of you if you ask for help, but not asking for help and getting into trouble is less easy to forgive.

Special situations require special solutions. You have to innovate, but you must be on the safe side and practice within the boundaries of your expertise. Read whatever you can to find out as much as possible about the subject. Somebody somewhere in the world must have faced the same problem. Today, with the internet, it is easier to get information. In this hospital, for the first time, we had a patient of purpura who underwent a laparoscopic splenectomy and a kidney transplant at the same sitting. This was probably a first in the world. The patient is alive and well and on the table. The platelet count did not fall below 7,000/dL and no blood or platelets were transfused. This was because of the input from various departments. One bag of platelets was arranged for and we had the help of a special analyzer machine, called a Thromboelastography (TEG). The spleen was removed laparoscopically and the transplant was done in the same sitting. Seeing the success of this case, another patient came to us for treatment along the same lines. Similarly, we had a patient who had purpura and was at full-term pregnancy. A cesarean section was planned, with the hematologist standing by. Today both mother and child are well and alive. Once you initiate something, others join in and people support each other, but you have to take as many people along as possible. Maybe not at this stage in your career, but later, you will have such opportunities.

Now, once you conceptualize what you are going to do and in which order, you have to visualize in your mind as if the operation is actually going on. Sit alone for 5 minutes and think. Even if it is a simple ingrown toenail, think about how you are going to tackle it. Are there any special instructions you need to give people? If you want only xylocaine, you must make it clear to the others that you want 2% xylocaine. You should let it be known that you do not want adrenaline mixed with xylocaine. Make it very clear. Even if you are going to inject somebody's hemorrhoids or injects somebody's veins, you must make it very clear what you are asking for, check it. All this is done in your mind, well before the procedure. So that you are clear what you are asking for. Think about and visualize any special position the patient will need to be placed in, any special requirement for the draping, and any special drugs the patient is on that you have to be cautious about or which you want to administer on the table. Think about it in your mind and visualize it. Simple mistakes are often made by the people who bring the instruments or clean them, prepare the drugs and drape the patient. Simple mistakes do happen. For example, the top of an insulin vial bears the number "40", in small print, denoting 40 units/mL. People sometimes mistakenly think that the whole bottle contains 40 units and inject the whole lot. Four hundred units gone straight into the patient's veins and then, to your surprise, the patient dies. For such reasons, too, you have to be very clear on what you are you dealing with and plan the procedure carefully.

Next, you have to plan the operation, the way one peels an onion layer by layer. Where will you make the incision and how long should it be? What will you find once you have made the incision? Where is the bleeding expected to be? Each area of the body has some well-defined veins or arteries, which you will come across. If you are performing a hernia operation, you will always run into a superficial epigastric vein. If you do not look for it, you will spend a good five minutes stopping the bleeding from that vein. Visualize the scenario, pause to look for the vein, tie it off and prevent it from bleeding. You now come to the next layer, and then the next. At each layer, you look for what you expect to find, until you finally come to the "problem" area. You define the problem, see the problem, and think of proceeding as planned. But it may happen that you suddenly come across a situation that is totally different from the one you had anticipated. For example, you think it is a tumor but it is actually a deep-seated abscess. You poke your finger into it and what comes out is pus or you go in thinking it is a cecal lump, but when you open the patient's abdomen, you find that it is an ovarian cyst. Before the operation, therefore, you should visualize how things can turn out to be different from what you are envisaging.

Such misdiagnoses should not occur in today's world, considering the number of modern investigative tools available. But they can occur and have occurred! Conceptualizing the surgery and planning beforehand entails a consideration of details such as: "I will make the first suture coming from this side"; "I will have the first tie come from this side"; "If the needle is in one direction, I will change the next one from the other direction"; "What will my assistant do in between, and how should arrange it?" You can almost bring it down to the last comma and full stop. It can always be done in any operation. When you watch any great surgeon, you will find that they make it look so easy. They never need to repeat anything. A limited number of gauze pieces, a limited number of movements. The same operation, the same monotonous manner, the regularity can become almost boring. But that is the mark of a great surgeon. In between, you must also check with the anesthetist. If you are going to make a cut and it is going to bleed, the anesthetist should be aware. In an adrenal tumor, for example, when you know that you are going to tie the adrenal vein, you must inform the anesthetist.

Imagining a situation beforehand is of great importance. Ask yourself: "What incision should I make? What is suitable for this patient? Will she be grateful if I give her a long midline or will she be grateful if I make it smaller?" Plan the number of packs that you may need, the sutures you have to use. Planning saves time. There are other things you can do to save time. A lot of time is spent on pointless effort.

Reducing bleeding is important. Some surgeons are hemorrhagic, while others are hemostatic! Some surgeons only have to touch a patient for the patient to start bleeding, while others may encounter the most horrifying bleeding and only have to put their hand on the spot for the bleeding to stop miraculously. So, what is the difference between their approaches? It is up to you to find out how some surgeons make the bleeding stop.

Another important point is knowing how to treat your assistant. Your assistant has not rushed to the operation theater (OT) in the morning to be abused by you. He/she has come with the desire to help you and expects to get a word of praise from you. Your assistant needs to be told what to do and it is up to you to tell him/her. Tell him/her what you want in advance. Be clear and repeat if needed! It is up to you to get the best out of your assistant.

Now, the single most important question: "Have I done enough?" What is wrong with the patient is not what matters. What matters is do you need to do something different surgically. If so, when? Do you need to do something immediately; Is the patient dying? Can you wait for an hour and convert it into a planned emergency? Can you wait for a week, for a month? What should you look for before closing the abdomen? You know, you are dealing with a malignancy somewhere, where should you be looking for it? There are hydatid cysts somewhere, should you look for them elsewhere? What else should you be looking for? Has the patient safely reversed from anesthesia at the end of surgery? All surgeons make this mistake. "The patient is fine. Okay, I am going." No! You have to make absolutely certain that the patient has been safely reversed. Always! Even if you have to leave the OT for some reason, get back to the OT on phone and confirm whether the patient has been reversed. It is the surgeon's responsibility. You have to ensure that the patient has been safely reversed. If not, where is the patient headed? Will the patient require to be transferred to an intensive care unit? Arrange for it in advance. Do not leave it to the anesthetist or anybody else. This is also a part of visualizing your operation.

Lastly, you must go out and tell the relatives what you have done. Never fudge, never try to hide what you have done. Be honest. People will accept it. How you express yourself is your business, but never try to duck and dive. This is one of the reasons why OTs throughout the world have only one door. There is no way that the surgeon can leave through the backdoor.

I have tried to outline a few points that may be helpful. Most of these are about thinking and planning beforehand. Now I come to the most basic requirement: knowledge. No surgeon should think that he/she is only a technician. A surgeon is a "learned technician". If you wish to be a surgeon, you must read. There are just a handful of books that all of us have read and grown with. Those books are all you require. They will never fail you. But you must read, and read again. Read before the operation to plan and immediately afterward to get confirmation. You may find that what you did was the only thing that could have been done or that you could have done it differently or in a better fashion. Because nothing is new, no matter what we think, it has all been done before, all has been seen before. It is all there in those two or three books which we need to know but you must read them both before and after surgery.

The best way of learning is observation. Watch how different people operate. Their technique may be different from what you learnt. Our system of teaching is not structured, the way the American system is. Though, to my mind, it is better to have a structured system—to be taught exactly how to hold a needle, how to tie knots, and so on. One can always evolve later. To get back to the point, watch many surgeons operate. There are many helpful videos available on the internet. They not only show all the steps, but also tell you about the technique. However, there are not as many videos on open surgeries as there are on laparoscopic surgeries.

So, Think! Read! and Observe! And do it once more before you operate.

Art of Assistance in Surgery: "Standing beside You"

Abha Majumdar

■ INTRODUCTION

Surgical assistants are important pillars of success in surgery. Not only do they enhance the competence and professionalism of the surgeon at the operation theater (OT) table but also make the surgeon comfortable. This makes a great contribution to the ultimate outcome of a surgery. Assistance is an art that is seldom discussed or taught. Assistants learn and improve as they go along and pick up the skills required to finally don the mantle of the lead surgeon. Let us discuss these skills in the following sections.

■ INCISION

An assistant is usually required to start a surgery by making an incision while the principal operator scrubs. To ensure ease of surgery, make sure that the incision is neither so big that triangles of tissue jut out from the retracted space nor so small as to reduce the visibility of the operating areas after the retractors are in place. In short, it should be of just the size that makes the surgeon comfortable during the surgery. Another thing you need to understand is that no matter how neat or beautiful a surgery is as regards the surgical skill, it matters little to the patient and her relatives if the incision scar is aesthetically displeasing. Hence, make an incision that is as straight and delicately drawn as the first line drawn by an artist on an expensive piece of canvas. This is even more true if the patient is a young child or a teenaged girl. An ugly scar is bound to dent her self-confidence. A lot of Indian women wear saris, so an abdominal incision should be made as low as possible. For those who wear skirts, scars on the legs should be as unobtrusive as possible.

■ RETRACTION

The position of the retractor is crucial in enabling the principal operator to have a good view of the surgical field and operate comfortably. Though it is not possible to list all the rules and norms related to different techniques for different procedures, a few tips may be helpful. There is a tendency among assistants to drop the handle of the retractor just above the skin level, so that her/his hand can rest over it. However, if the retractor is held in this position, the operating space is reduced as the retractor blade is at right angles with the handle. Raising the handle so that it is at a 30° with the skin allows the retracting blade to move inward, thus increasing the visual and working area of surgery. To do this comfortably, you need to hold the distal end of the retractor so that you do not have to raise your hand very high in order not to interfere with the main surgeon's movement. Remember that retraction does not mean forceful separation of the skin and fascial edges. Gentle retraction not only reduces tissue trauma and postoperative pain but also reduces the assistant's fatigue to a great extent.

■ BLEEDERS

While operating, if you come upon a "spurter", do not jump to put a sponge on it to press it down immediately. The best way to catch a bleeder is while it is still spurting. It stops spurting after a few seconds and if you do not catch it within that time, you need to dab it and compress it, and then remove or roll the sponge gradually to see it bleed and catch it. If the bleeding is so profuse that it conceals the bleeder from your vision, it may not be possible to pass the stitch around the vessel to ligate it. Then you need to suction all around the area with active bleeding, keeping the suction about half a centimeter away from the area filling fastest with blood, to enable the surgeon to pass a stitch more easily and faster to ligate the bleeder. Please use a needle holder rather than artery forceps if you are required to assist the surgeon in pulling out the needle from its tip. If artery forceps are used to hold the needle, they may develop irregular spicules, which then tend to damage or break the suture material that they are supposed to hold. You may use metal clips to stop bleeding vessels that are extremely difficult to ligate.

■ HOLDING A CLAMP

After clamping and cutting tissue which has vessels in it, avoid holding the clamp such that the tip is low and the proximal part is higher. The best way to hold a clamp is to raise the tip a little to make more tissue available distally, giving the surgeon more space to pass the ligature and minimizing the risk of ligature slipping. Do not use artery forceps and Allis forceps to hold tissue unnecessarily and refrain from pulling rashly upon tissue, since tissue injury and the formation of microhematomas cause postoperative pain. To summarize, be kind to tissue and handle it gently.

To conclude, a competent assistant is he who knows the operation well and can assist to enhance the efficacy of the surgeon.

CHAPTER

7

The Art of Selecting a Suitable Incision in Surgery and Art of Retraction

Vijay Arora

■ INTRODUCTION

Incisions are linear cuts made in the skin and deepened by cutting through layers of tissue to reach the site of pathology and planned operative procedure. The incision allows access to the area (e.g., abdomen or thorax) where the intended surgical procedure is to be carried out.

■ PRINCIPLES OF MAKING INCISIONS

- *Skin incisions*: These should follow Langer's lines.
- *Accessibility*: An incision must allow the surgeon to reach the organ of interest. Its placement may be directly over the organ or in accordance with a planned route of deepening the incision.
- *Least damage en route*: An incision must be planned in such a way as to avoid injury to vessels, nerves or other important structures, which must be identified, separated and protected. In a thoracotomy, for example, the intercostal incision is made in such a way as to avoid injury to the intercostal neurovascular bundle.
- *Deepening an incision*: This may require muscles to be cut, however, most incisions are planned so as to split muscles where possible and avoid cutting. The classic example is McBurney's incision, where all muscles are split, even though they are at right angles to each other, till the peritoneum is reached.
- *Extensibility*: The length of an incision may need to be increased depending on the area which has to be accessed for the surgical procedure. Making an incision that does not allow for extension may require the surgeon to make another incision.
- *Security*: An incision must be closed such that on healing, it secures the operated area and is not prone to complications, particularly incisional hernia.
- *Abdominal surgery*: The preferred approach is to use vertical incisions.
  - *Midline incision*: This is the most commonly used incision. It passes through the linea alba after the skin and is almost bloodless with no nerves or vessels encountered. It is the most extensible incision that can be taken from the xiphisternum to the symphysis pubis—encircling or through the umbilicus. It allows access to all intra-abdominal and retroperitoneal structures and can be closed quickly.
  - *Paramedian incision*: This is made with the rectus muscles being retracted and is supposed to be more secure. However, there are greater chances of incisional hernia as the rectus muscle may weaken due to traction on the neurovascular supply. It is also

more time consuming to make and close it. Besides, the opposite side of the abdomen is not easily accessible. Oblique or transverse incisions are preferred because they allow access to the desired area.

- *Kocher's incision*: This is subcostally placed and oblique on either side for approach to the upper abdominal viscera. It is an extendible incision and both sides may be joined for the chevron (rooftop), bucket-handle or Mercedes Benz modifications.
- *Midabdomen transverse muscle-cutting incision*: This is commonly used for laparotomy in newborns and infants as the length of vertical incision is limited. It is also preferred in short and obese adults. Being a muscle-cutting incision, there is the possibility of incisional hernia formation.
- *McBurney's incision*: This is the classic muscle-splitting incision for appendicectomy. It may be modified by changing the direction of the skin cut to transverse (Lanz). It is extensible and when made muscle-cutting, as in the Rutherford–Morrison modification, allows for right- or left-sided colonic resection.
- *Lower abdominal transverse incision*: It is described by Pfannenstiel, this is used extensively by gynecologists and pelvic surgeons. It heals very well and is a secure incision.
- *Thoracic incisions*: These are mostly intercostal and are made to approach the lungs and esophagus. The preferred cardiac incision is the median sternotomy in which the sternum is cut along the midline and retracted. Bone closure requires wire sutures.
- *Thoracoabdominal incisions*: These are extended, intercostal incisions on the abdominal wall, made in an oblique fashion, usually through the 5th to the 7th intercostal space. This allows access to both the pleural and peritoneal cavities at the same time. These are used in hepatic surgery and surgery of the esophagus/stomach.
- *Breast surgery incisions*: These are made radial to avoid cutting the milk ducts or circumareolar skin incisions deepened by radial incision in the breast tissue. The classic radical mastectomy incision described by Halsted, runs from the shoulder to the xiphisternum obliquely, but now many modifications, mostly transverse, have been adopted. Inframammary incisions are sometimes used to avoid making incisions through the breast tissue.
- *Neck surgery incisions*: Transverse or oblique incisions are required for operation on the thyroid and salivary glands. Neck dissection in a radical operation for head/neck malignancy needs to be tailored to suit the specific requirement.
- *Inguinal incision*: This is designed specifically for inguinal hernia repair; this is an oblique incision running parallel to the inguinal ligament.

The choice of incision is dependent on many factors including the surgeon's experience and training. Some of these factors are:

- Organ to be operated upon
- Extent of surgery radicality
- Need for stoma placement
- Whether speed is essential—midline incision in exploratory laparotomy
- Built of the patient
- Degree of obesity

- Previous incisions—it is preferable to enter the abdomen through a virgin area, but the old scar may need to be excised and then careful dissection carried out to avoid injury to underlying structures, which may be adherent.

PRINCIPLES OF WOUND CLOSURE

- Handle tissue gently
- Ensure hemostasis
- Eliminate tension as it leads to impaired healing and bad scars. The use of relaxing incision has been described and flap mobilization may be necessary to close the wound.
- Evert wound edges
- Respect Langer's lines and skin folds when closing
- If crossing a joint, place oblique, or transverse incision
- Closure in layers is the norm, but the technique of mass closure of large wounds is often employed. In the closure of a laparotomy incision, three-layered closure using catgut is no longer in vogue. A two-layered closure is employed—peritoneum, muscle, and fascia with a continuous loop suture using delayed absorbable suture; and skin with subcutaneous fat as the second layer. It may be required to leave the skin open for a delayed primary closure or secondary closure in patients with peritonitis.

ESSENTIALS OF RETRACTION

Retraction is the art of pulling and counter-pulling the wound edges to allow the surgeon to visualize an organ and approach a distant structure.

It is best if both the surgeon and the assistant can see the structure in question, but it is essential that the retraction allows the surgeon to have an unhindered view.

- The pulls can be used intelligently in various directions. The fulcrum is at the wound edge and allows the traction to get to deeper areas.
- Retractors are designed for a particular job and should be selected carefully (**Fig. 1**). There are specifically designed retractors for vessels, nerves, and lungs.
- Retractors are available in varying sizes to allow small wound edges retraction to retract the liver lobes.
- Malleable retractors allow contour modification
- Self-retaining retractors allow the assisting surgeon to use her/his hands to assist the principal surgeon

INCISIONS IN LAPAROSCOPIC SURGERY

The development of laparoscopy made the surgical approach to various organs radically different from conventional open surgery. By making the incision smaller, laparoscopy reduced the trauma of access. Hence, it is now described as minimal access surgery.

The incisions are usually 3–12 mm in size and are all muscle splitting. Their placement is planned keeping in view the ergometrics of approach where the incision is placed far away from the area of interest. In laparoscopic appendectomy, for example, the instruments are passed from the left flank or midline.

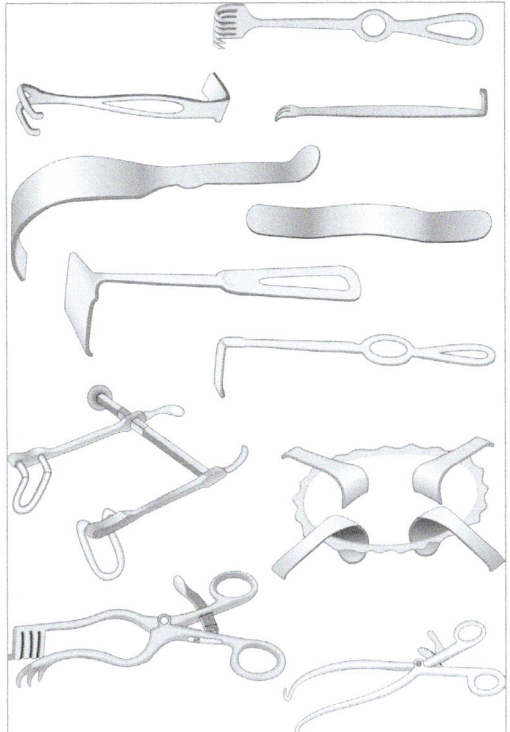

Fig. 1: Various retractors in surgery.

The closure of incisions of up to 5 mm does not need any suture except skin. Larger incisions need to be closed using devices such as wound closure needles used in a mass closure, e.g., Endo Close™ (Medtronic, USA) and port closure needles.

Incisions of 2 cm are used in single-incision minimal access surgery. These require proper layered closure and are prone to the same complications as incisions in conventional surgery.

■ POSTOPERATIVE COMPLICATIONS

- Postoperative pain is less in transverse incisions than in vertical incisions.
- Wound infections depend on the disease, whether the surgery is planned or emergency, involvement of bowel surgery, and patient risk factors such as being immunocompromised and having coexisting sepsis. No significant difference in infections rates among the different types of incision or the techniques have been reported.
- Source of infection may be contamination from the external or internal environment.
- Wound dehiscence rate is higher in vertical incisions than in transverse or oblique incisions.
- Incisional hernia has been reported in 2–20% of patients after abdominal incisions. The factors influencing incisional hernia are wound healing or its delay, wound infection, patient immunocompetence, diabetes mellitus, obesity, age and emergency surgery. The rate of incisional hernia is higher in vertical incisions than in transverse or oblique incisions.

Approach to a Lady as a Surgical Patient

Abha Majumdar

■ INTRODUCTION

This section deals with an important aspect of treating a female patient surgically, that is, the approach to be adopted toward surgery for female patients.

■ RULE OUT PREGNANCY

Before operating on a female patient, you must rule out pregnancy. If the woman has missed her period or if a reliable history cannot be elicited, you should carry out at least one available confirmatory test, such as the urine pregnancy test, serum beta-human chorionic gonadotropin (β-hCG) or ultrasound examination. This is essential for the preoperative decision regarding the surgical methods to be used. Further, pregnancy may necessitate a change in the line of treatment.

■ ORAL CONTRACEPTIVE PILLS OR HORMONE REPLACEMENT THERAPY

You should confirm whether the woman is on oral contraceptive pills (OCPs). This is important because most women do not consider these medicines and tend not to mention them when giving their medical history. Women on OCPs, those who have taken a morning-after pill in the preceding few days and elderly women on hormone replacement therapy are all at a higher risk of thromboembolism, especially if they also smoke or are obese. If you fear that the woman has deep vein thrombosis, using perioperative anticoagulants, earlier mobilization, elevation, and exercising the limbs as soon after surgery as possible are the preferable treatment options.

■ RESPECT FOR PRIVACY

Make sure that when your patient walks into the operation theater (OT), she is wearing proper slippers and clothes that are not falling off or opening out from all sides. Similarly, see to it that she is covered by a proper sheet or blanket when she is being wheeled in. A lack of respect is very embarrassing for the patient who is, as it is, nervous about the surgery and may lower her self-esteem and confidence. Similarly, when a patient is being wheeled out of the OT or her relatives are called in to see her, you must ensure that she is covered properly and is in a comfortable position before she wakes up.

Another important point you must remember is to make sure that the technicians do not start pulling her gown or clothes for the purpose of placing the electrocardiogram (ECG) leads or start placing her in positions other than the supine position, in which she is lying while still awake. It is equally important not to uncover her while deciding on the incision lines before anesthesia. Also, while taking care of these minor details, you would do better not to sit over your patient like a hawk, as this may have a permanently adverse effect on her experience of surgery.

A daily situation faced in obstetric practice is when a pregnant woman or patient in labor is taken up for epidural or spinal anesthesia or analgesia. Her gown either needs to be opened wide or raised to her upper waist to allow for easy access to the area for regional injection. Make sure you use an additional sheet to cover the lower part of her body. The same goes for catheterizing a patient or putting her in a lithotomy position before administering general anesthesia or epidural/spinal anesthesia while she is still awake. Procedures such as covering the patient well will preserve her sense of dignity. These rules need to be followed more precisely when the patient is a hospital staff member as she is familiar with the people around her in the OT.

■ CHECKLIST OF PROCEDURES AND SIDE OF OPERATION

As in the case of other procedures, you should make sure that the right patient has been wheeled in, the right surgery has been written and confirmed, and the correct side noted before surgery. Time and time again the principal surgeon has had to face criminal litigation because the standard operating protocol was either not defined or not followed by his team.

■ TYPE OF ANESTHESIA

It is of the utmost importance for surgeons and their assistants to discuss with the anesthetists the best method of anesthesia for their patient, especially if she is pregnant, and also inform her before administering it. In case the patient is not comfortable with the method of anesthesia, there should be an alternative method available that does not compromise her or the unborn child's well-being.

■ POSITION OF THE PATIENT

An assistant needs to know this thoroughly as he is the one who initiates the surgery. If the surgery is to be in a dorsal position, then for women who are about to have a cesarean section, the position of the head (how low) plus the lateral tilts need to be taken care of. As for lithotomy positions, it is very important for every assistant to know how low or high or how flexed or extended the thighs need to be, or how wide apart the legs should be placed to facilitate surgery.

■ SURGERIES WITH PSYCHOLOGICAL IMPACT

An extra word of caution is required for operations that affect the patient's idea of womanhood. You must talk to the patient about the fact that she will have to shave her head a day before a head surgery requiring craniotomy. If the patient is not informed and mentally prepared beforehand, it may come as a shock and prove to be traumatic. In the case of a colostomy or urostomy, you should sit with the husband and wife and tell them about the implications of the procedure, which would also affect their sex lives. Certain surgeries, such as mastectomy, may have an immense psychological impact, and it is important to deal with the patient very gently. You may need to take the help of the patient's near and dear ones to prepare her for such surgical procedures. Unlike mastectomy, hysterectomy has less of a psychological impact because it does not change the patient's appearance and thus does not lower her self-esteem. With mastectomy, which may have a devastating effect on her, a lot of preprocedure and postoperative counseling is essential.

■ ELDERLY PATIENTS

Here, three important things need to be considered: (1) you may seem too young to the patient, (2) an elderly patient may be relatively more reserved when discussing her problems, and (3) the patient's bones are likely to be more brittle than those of other age groups. If you do not handle the patient carefully when positioning her, especially when she is under anesthesia, she is more likely than others to suffer a fracture. In general, you must treat these patients with the dignity they deserve.

Lastly, no surgery should be postponed only because a patient is menstruating. In these situations, the nursing staff may need to act with a little more tact than usual.

Approach to a Child as a Surgical Patient

Anurag Krishna

■ INTRODUCTION

Operations have been performed on children for many centuries but it was only around 1914 that the specialty of pediatric surgery was developed, as a result of a major shipwreck off the coast of Canada. People believed that there was a need to create this specialty because the handling and treatment of children should be different from those of adults. This arose from the knowledge that the physiology, pharmacology and pharmacokinetics in the case of children were quite different from those in the case of adults. Initially, vague calculations were made to determine the dose of medications for children, going by body weight, e.g., they may have been given one-fifth of the dose given to an adult. However, realization dawned with the occurrence of a major disaster, in which a lot of children became trauma victims. The purpose of creating the specialty of pediatric surgery was not merely to create a select group of doctors to treat children, but to set standards of surgical care for children.

Let us consider a situation in which a preterm baby weighing 1.5 kg has to undergo a surgery within a couple of hours of birth. Your job is not only to treat the medical condition of the baby, but to handle the anxiety of the child as well as that of the family. So, anxiety management is an integral part of the overall management of children. The second problem is communication. It is often said that treating children is like veterinary surgery because like animals, children cannot verbalize or vocalize their problems. However, they have their own subtle and not-so-subtle ways of communicating exactly what the problem is. It is up to you to be able to detect these signals. I remember when I was an intern, the moment I would approach a child to examine him/her, the child would start shouting. My initial response would be to frown at the helpless child who was not settling down. This is a natural reaction, but you should be able to develop the ability to handle a child.

The third big worry is that babies have very poor reserves. They are walking on a thin line. Anything can tip the balance of their physiology in an adverse manner, but on the other hand, if you handle them properly they bounce back quite fast. Obstetricians often face situations in which the baby does not cry after birth and turns blue, leading to panic, but quite suddenly, the first breath makes the baby cry, its color changes from blue to red and there is joy. So, you need to manage the critical balance very, very carefully. What children often need is a little support. Gentleness is of paramount importance, not only in the way you communicate with and handle a child, but also in the way you wield the knife. Gentle handling is equivalent to assured success. If you are rough in the handling of the case at any point, you are asking for trouble and making the task much more difficult for yourself.

Let us now take a short virtual walk through the operation theater. Many times, we omit, ignore or fail to think of simple things, considering them irrelevant, but this can be rectified with a slight change in approach. Imagine that you are in the preanesthetic room. The mother is holding the baby. Someone calls for the child, and a man trots up to the mother and grabs the child. The child cries and wails as he is taken down the corridor, after which he is dumped on the operating table. Many things have gone wrong.

One thing of primary importance that we omit is to keep the baby warm. Little babies do not have efficient thermoregulatory mechanisms. Very little attention is paid to this aspect in most operation theaters. For example, when dealing with a child who has suffered a trauma, in our attempt to see to his wounds, we uncover him completely. Our first reaction is to deal with the internal bleeding as fast as possible. As a result, the bleeding may get controlled within 10–15 minutes of the laparotomy, but the child may now have hypothermia. Hypothermia causes several severe metabolic derailment and it takes many hours, if not days, to sort them out. So, enough attention must be paid to keeping the child warm, whether you are seeing him in your examination room, the causality ward or the operation theater.

In addition, it is of critical importance to ensure that the air passages are not blocked. A child's air passages are extremely tiny and compromised. A child may stop breathing if respiration is obstructed by any small plug somewhere, secretions, his own vomit, etc. You must be extremely prompt in dealing with such a situation.

The blood volume of a child weighing 1.5 kg would be 80–100 mL/kg. So, we are talking about 120–150 mL of blood. If a child loses 15 mL of blood, he has lost 10% of the blood volume, which qualifies him for blood replacement. You must not forget that maintaining the blood volume is of paramount importance. But that is not all; the right proportion has to be kept in mind in many instances. For example, it would be all right if you soaked four gauze pieces in the case of a 40-year-old patient with a hernia, but you would be in trouble if you do the same in the case of a child.

Children do not give you much time or too many chances.

You should deal with them quickly and efficiently, and try to get it right in the first go. You must not dilly-dally while making decisions, or it may be too late. Reading, practicing, and observing how people handle and treat children are probably the best ways of learning for how to approach a child in the surgery.

One aspect we tend to ignore is handling a child gently and carefully. In England, pediatric wards are very cheerful. The nurses do not wear uniforms, but bright and cheerful dresses. Their hair is decked with small, colorful ribbons. A consultant, no matter how stiff his joints, bends down on his knees and plays with the child, especially when he is going to operate on the child. Being on the same physical level as the child helps to gain his confidence. You have to physically come down to his level because he cannot come up to you. Playing with the child and his toys also helps to gain his trust. Examining the child and being with him will tell you far more than what his parents say or what you have read in textbooks. The disease is written on the child's face." A child does not lie! If he says, "It hurts here," it means it does hurt "here". But you have to get him to tell you where it hurts. So you need to spend a few minutes with him. You, therefore, have to cultivate the right attitude.

Pain—Friend or Foe

Pradeep Jain, Naresh Dua

■ INTRODUCTION

Pain is defined as "an unpleasant sensory or emotional experience associated with actual or potential tissue damage, or described in terms of such damage." It acts as both friend and foe.

Pain whether friend or foe, is transmitted in a similar manner to the brain. The line that separates the two is very thin, linked to the duration, intensity, cause, and social and economic factors that affect the ability to endure and fight pain.

Any stimulus that is damaging to the tissues, stimulates the nociceptors in the periphery and then is transmitted to the spinal cord and brain, leading to the perception of pain as well as triggering of motor and autonomic reflexes to prevent damage and help in healing. If the intensity of the stimulus is prolonged, there is sensitization of the system, leading to enhanced excitability termed hyperalgesia. In hyperalgesia, pain serves a protective function by decreasing the mobility and function of the affected part until healing takes place.

When pain is triggered by irrelevant, inappropriate or prolonged stimulus or a stimulus of exaggerated intensity due to the dysfunction or disease of the peripheral or central nervous system, the normal relationship between pain and injury is breached and pain becomes the enemy: very difficult to treat, distressful, a burden on the patient and society.

■ PAIN AS A FRIEND

Pain is a neurological response to a situation which stimulates the brain to trigger autonomic and motor reflexes to save the body from impending damage. Pain is not a disease. It is a symptom of imminent damage. For example, when we touch a hot plate, our body's autonomic reflex generated by the pain mechanism makes us move away very quickly so as to prevent a burn injury. Thus, pain is merely a symptom, and finding the cause of pain is the key to protecting the body from further harm.

As an example, let us consider a headache, a pain that arises from the head or upper neck and originates from tissues and structures that surround the skull or brain. It is a symptom of medical issues such as sinusitis, eye problems, vascular disorders of the brain and spinal cord, meningitis, substance abuse, and withdrawal. In any of these, treating just the headache would not cure the underlying condition. Thus, a headache is a valuable warning signal of a pathological process, demanding action to diagnose and treat the underlying cause. For this reason, in ancient times, pain was described as the "barking watchdog of health".

Suppression of pain could, in fact, be dangerous. In peripheral diabetic neuropathy, for example, raised blood glucose levels and triglycerides cause microvascular injury, damaging nerve fibers and leading to the loss of the protective sensations of touch, temperature and pain, so the feedback mechanism of the body that generates motor and autonomic responses to protect itself is also lost. Thus, minor injuries caused by walking around barefoot, or injury by sharp objects, or due to friction with ill-fitting shoes may go unnoticed and ultimately result in severe infection or foot ulcers. The loss of the sensation of pain in autonomic diabetic neuropathy accounts for silent myocardial infarction, which delays treatment and may result in a fatal outcome.

Leprosy is another disease that is associated with nontraumatic neuropathy with functional derangement of peripheral nerves. The earliest sensory involvement in leprosy is the inability to discriminate between heat and cold. This is followed by the loss of the sensation of touch and then the sensation of pain, leading to minor injuries, breaks or burns being unnoticed and later getting infected or turning into more critical problems, such as trophic ulcers, Charcot's joints or mutilations.

■ PAIN AS A FOE

Though pain is generally a friend, it may sometimes become a foe. This happens when pain becomes chronic and dissociated from the original pathological process causing it. As a result, the sufferer is no longer in a position to switch it off like an alarm bell. A cautioning friend then becomes an intolerable burden. This occurs because of increased central sensitization of low-threshold tactile afferents in the nociceptive pathway, which causes the registration of chronic pain in the limbic system (cerebral pain center) to intensify. A vicious cycle results, which if not broken, is detrimental to the patient and society. Let us consider three case scenarios.

Case I: A 56-year-old male presented with a history of moderate to severe pain in the right T8-T10 dermatomes since 3 years. Pain occurred with touch or even the movement of air. He had suffered from herpes zoster infection in the same region 3 years earlier. He had been treated with acyclovir and analgesics at that time, but the pain did not dissipate. Thereafter, he was treated with a variety of medications, including gabapentin, nortriptyline, 5% lidocaine patch, but with no relief. This tactile allodynia (postherpetic neuralgia) caused by the reactivation of the varicella zoster virus and damage to the sensory neurons became a disease.

Case II: A 60-year-old male with a history of heavy smoking presented with severe pain in the left leg since 2 years. He had been diagnosed with peripheral vascular disease after a Doppler study and had undergone a left femoropopliteal bypass a year after the start of pain. Six months after the bypass surgery, he presented with severe pain in the left leg and early signs of gangrene. The bypass was found to be occluded, and treatment with medicines for 2 months was unsuccessful, so the left foot was amputated. The pain abated for 2 weeks but then reappeared and gradually worsened. The symptoms were continuous and described as aching, tightening, and burning. The patient was diagnosed with phantom limb pain.

Case III: A 62-year-old male presented with severe pain and muscular spasms in the left leg and foot. He had a history of poorly controlled diabetes mellitus, hypertension, and a minor stroke 6 months earlier that had caused numbness in his left extremities. The numbness gradually developed into a tingling sensation and then increased to pain on touch: the poststroke pain.

■ CONCLUSION

Pain therefore, although a protective mechanism that warns of an impending damage may also be an unnecessary burden that causes a huge psychological effect and may need appropriate management to relieve the patient of this unpleasant experience.

■ SUGGESTED READING

1. Cervero F. Pain: friend or foe? A Neurobiologic perspective: the 2008 Bonica Award Lecture. Reg Anesth Pain Med. 2009;34:569-74.
2. Dyck PJB, Sinnreich M. Diabetic Neuropathies. Continuum. 2003;9:19-34.
3. Hunt SP, Mantyh PW. The molecular dynamics of pain control. Nat Rev Neurosci. 2001;2:83-91.
4. Kar S, Krishnan A, Singh N, Singh R, Pawar S. Nerve damage in leprosy: An electrophysiological evaluation of ulnar and median nerves in patients with clinical neural deficits: A pilot study. Indian Dermatol Online J. 2013;4:97-101.
5. Klein T, Magerl W, Rolke R, Treede RD. Human surrogate models of neuropathic pain. Pain. 2005;115:227-33.
6. Levitt NS, Stansberry KB, Wynchank S, Vinik AI. The natural progression of autonomic neuropathy and autonomic function tests in a cohort of people with IDDM. Diabetes Care. 1996;19:751-4.
7. Rathmann W, Ziegler D, Jahnke M, Haastert B, Gries FA. Mortality in diabetic patients with cardiovascular autonomic neuropathy. Diabet Med. 1993;10:820-4.
8. Smith WC, Anderson AM, Withington SG, van Brakel WH, Croft RP, Nicholls PG, et al. Steroid prophylaxis for prevention of nerve function impairment in leprosy: Randomised placebo controlled trial (TRIPOD 1). BMJ. 2004;328:1459.
9. Treede RD, Meyer RA, Raja SN, Campbell JN. Peripheral and central mechanisms of cutaneous hyperalgesia. Prog Neurobiol. 1992;38:397-421.
10. Whitesides TE Jr. Pain: friend or foe? J Bone Joint Surg Am. 2001;83:1424-5.
11. Woolf CJ, Salter MW. Neuronal plasticity: Increasing the gain in pain. Science. 2000; 288:1765-9.

Progress in Minimal Access Surgery

Vivek Bindal, Anupam Goel

■ HISTORY

Minimal access surgery (MAS) has had a huge impact on the way surgery has been practiced in the last few decades. It started in 1901 with an experimental laparoscopy, called celioscopy, performed on a dog by George Kelling, using a Nitze cystoscope. In 1910, Jacobeus performed the first human thoracoscopic diagnosis of tuberculosis using a cystoscope, and also the first human celioscopy. To ensure safe insertion and for insufflation of the peritoneal cavity, a needle with a spring-loaded obturator was developed by Veress in 1938. Forestier introduced illumination by fiberoptic technology, which allowed for bright illumination without the risk of burns. In 1953, Harold Hopkins introduced the Hopkins rod—lens system, which improved clarity and illuminance by >80 times.

In 1982, Kurt Semm, the German gynecologist, performed the first laparoscopic appendectomy. The first human laparoscopic cholecystectomy was performed in 1987 by the French surgeon, Philippe Mouret, using four trocars. McKernan and Saye performed the first laparoscopic cholecystectomy in the United States in 1988, but the technique was refined and popularized by Reddick and Olsen. In 1991, Tay and Smoot developed intraperitoneal onlay mesh repair, which is effective for smaller defects. For inguinal hernia repair, Arregui and Dion reported the first trans-abdominal preperitoneal repair in 1993, while McKernon and Laws reported the first (total extraperitoneal repair the same year).

■ TECHNOLOGICAL ADVANCES

Imaging

Technology has played a major role in the journey from basic laparoscopy, practiced in the 1980s and early 1990s, to advanced laparoscopic procedures. Earlier, the surgeon's posture was usually not appropriate as he would use one hand to look directly into the endoscope and perform the surgery with his other hand. One of the major advancements in MAS was the development of a video computer chip that allowed for the magnification and projection of images onto television screens. With this, the techniques of laparoscopic surgery truly became integrated into the discipline of general surgery. Now, the exposure of the operative field by the assistant, using the imaging system, became possible, while the surgeon could perform the procedure using both his hands. The surgeon's posture became more normal, causing less fatigue, and resulting in better ergonomics. This advancement also helped in the dissemination of surgical techniques by observation, video recording, and the transmission of surgical videos to a large number of surgeons.

The quality of images has improved over the last two decades from standard definition to high-definition imaging systems. This technology is ever changing, what with the evolution of 4K, 3D, and fluorescence imaging. A good imaging system is a prerequisite for the development of more advanced procedures in the field of MAS.

Fluorescence techniques in minimally invasive surgery make it possible to visualize features that are invisible under conventional white light. The use of near-infrared imaging with indocyanine green (ICG) dye has expanded the spectrum of diagnostic options and made the perfusion evaluation of organs and tissues possible. It also helps in visualizing hepatic lesions and the biliary anatomy as ICG dye is secreted by hepatocytes. It is helpful in identifying sentinel lymph nodes in patients with malignancy. Narrow-band imaging endoscopy is a technology that enhances optical images and allows for a detailed inspection of vascular and mucosal patterns, enabling the surgeon to predict histology during real-time endoscopy or laparoscopy.

Electrosurgery

Electrosurgery has evolved over the decades from the use of monopolar and traditional bipolar to advanced bipolar and ultrasonic energy sources. Monopolar cautery can both cut and coagulate, but the lateral thermal spread is relatively greater, it produces smoke and charring, and the grounding plate has to be remote from the site of surgery. Traditional bipolar cautery only coagulates and the grounding prong is close to the active prong at the surgical site, which prevents the flow of current from the patient's body.

The modern electrosurgical units incorporate sophisticated microprocessors and feedback systems that monitor impedance (resistance) and/or temperature. The unit automatically adjusts the delivery of radiofrequency electrical energy in order to ensure adequate tissue sealing. Advanced bipolar devices can both cut and coagulate the tissue with minimal thermal spread and a better ability to seal vessels.

Ultrasonic energy devices convert electrical energy to mechanical energy. An active jaw oscillates in a linear fashion at a frequency of 23–55 kHz over the tissue against a passive articulated jaw, producing a mechanical friction. Ultrasonic energy devices can both cut and coagulate tissue with minimal lateral thermal spread, decreased smoke production and better ability to seal vessels, and without the passage of current through the patient's body. The cavitron ultrasonic surgical aspirator, an innovative tool for dissecting the liver parenchyma, allows for simultaneous fragmenting, suction, and irrigation. It can potentially decrease intraoperative blood loss and perioperative morbidity.

These advanced electrosurgical units have made advanced MAS procedures feasible, decreasing surgical time, and achieving better hemostasis.

Ancillary Equipment

The latest carbon dioxide insufflators are high-flow insufflators which prevent a sudden decrease in intra-abdominal pressure due to the leakage of gases or excessive use of suction cannulas. Insufflators with a mechanism for temperature control help to prevent hypothermia, especially in long surgeries.

New laparoscopic hand instruments have been designed for needle laparoscopy and single port surgeries. These include bent and articulating instruments. Laparoscopy lacks the benefit of tactile stimulation, which has been overcome by the development of hand ports that allow the surgeon to put his hand inside the patient's abdomen while preventing the leakage of gases. This is especially useful in malignancy, large-sized masses, and hemorrhage.

There is a growing trend in favor of the use of disposable plastic trocars instead of metallic ones. The use of disposable trocars, though less cost-effective, has decreased the rate of traumatic and thermal injuries to the abdomen. Optical trocars help the surgeon to enter the abdomen under vision, which can prevent inadvertent vascular or visceral abdominal injury.

The advancements in endoscopic gastrointestinal anastomotic staplers have revolutionized minimally invasive management of gastrointestinal, oncological, and bariatric patients. These staplers can be used to transect vessels or gastrointestinal tissues and create gastrointestinal anastomosis with low leak and bleeding rates and shorter surgical time.

The set-up of the operating room (OR) has changed over the last decade to make MAS more comfortable. To prevent cluttering of equipment and the presence of wires on the ground, a wall-mounted set-up is preferred. The new OR tables can bear more weight and automatic control allows for better patient posture. Modular ORs with laminar air flow help reduce the infection rates.

Advances in Skill Set

Over the last two decades, training in MAS has improved due to well-structured fellowship programs, which enable trainees to perform mentored surgery, with decreasing complication rates. The availability of simulation laboratories, wet laboratories, endotrainers, and various MAS training programs has led to the spread of knowledge and skill set to a wide number of surgeons. The establishment of professional societies in the field of MAS has resulted in the development of definite guidelines and algorithms for various diseases, and the organization of continued medical education and training programs. This helps young surgeons to develop an adequate skill set.

Robotic Surgery

The latest development in the field of MAS is the robotic platform. It essentially consists of computer-assisted navigation with no artificial intelligence. It provides a digital interface between the surgeon and the patient. The advantages include three-dimensional vision, more degrees of freedom, improved dexterity, elimination of the fulcrum effect and tremor, and greater telesurgical capability and comfort for the surgeon.

Robotic instruments provide seven degrees of freedom, as against laparoscopy, which provides only five. Robotic surgery is especially useful in the case of the thorax and deep cavities of the abdomen, such as for retroperitoneal, pelvic, and upper gastrointestinal surgeries. The disadvantages of robotic surgery include its high cost, the learning curve, longer operating time, rapidly changing fields, and loss of haptic (tactile) sensation.

Benefit to Patients

Minimal access surgery has become more popular than open surgery because of better recovery after surgery, less postoperative pain, shorter hospital stay, and superior cosmesis. Further progress is being made toward reduced port, single port, and natural orifice surgeries. The development of robotics and artificial intelligence in the field of MAS holds a lot of promise for the future.

▋ SUGGESTED READING

1. Bindal V, Bhatia P, Dudeja U, Kalhan S, Khetan M, John S, et al. Review of contemporary role of robotics in bariatric surgery. J Minim Access Surg. 2015;11:16-21.
2. Boni L, David G, Mangano A, Dionigi G, Rausei S, Spampatti S, et al. Clinical applications of indocyanine green (ICG) enhanced fluorescence in laparoscopic surgery. Surg Endosc. 2015;29:2046-55.
3. Cuschieri A. Minimal access surgery and the future of interventional laparoscopy. Am J Surg. 1991;161:404-7.
4. Daskalakis M, Scheffel O, Weiner RA. High flow insufflation for the maintenance of the pneumoperitoneum during bariatric surgery. Obes Facts. 2009;2 Suppl 1(Suppl 1):37-40.
5. Jakimowicz JJ, Cuschieri A. Time for evidence-based minimal access surgery training—simulate or sink. Surg Endosc. 2005;19:1521-2.
6. Kelley WE Jr. The evolution of laparoscopy and the revolution in surgery in the decade of the 1990s. JSLS. 2008;12:351-7.
7. Kim JJ, Song KY, Chin HM, Kim W, Jeon HM, Park CH, et al. Totally laparoscopic gastrectomy with various types of intracorporeal anastomosis using laparoscopic linear staplers: Preliminary experience. Surg Endosc. 2008;22:436-42.
8. Landman J, Kerbl K, Rehman J, Andreoni C, Humphrey PA, Collyer W, et al. Evaluation of a vessel sealing system, bipolar electrosurgery, harmonic scalpel, titanium clips, endoscopic gastrointestinal anastomosis vascular staples and sutures for arterial and venous ligation in a porcine model. J Urol. 2003;169:697-700.
9. Lee SJ, Park KH. Ultrasonic energy in endoscopic surgery. Yonsei Med J. 1999; 40:545-9.
10. Oshinsky GS, Smith AD. Laparoscopic needles and trocars: An overview of designs and complications. J Laparoendosc Surg. 1992;2:117-25.
11. Reijnen MM, Zeebregts CJ, Meijerink WJ. Future of operating rooms. Surg Technol Int. 2005;14:21-7.
12. Sharma P, Bansal A, Mathur S, Wani S, Cherian R, McGregor D, et al. The utility of a novel narrow-band imaging endoscopy system in patients with Barrett's esophagus. Gastrointest Endosc. 2006;64:167-75.
13. Spaner SJ, Warnock GL. A brief history of endoscopy, laparoscopy, and laparoscopic surgery. J Laparoendosc Adv Surg Tech A. 1997;7:369-73.
14. van Bergen P, Kunert W, Buess GF. The effect of high-definition imaging on surgical task efficiency in minimally invasive surgery: An experimental comparison between three-dimensional imaging and direct vision through a stereoscopic TEM rectoscope. Surg Endosc. 2000;14:71-4.
15. Vecchio R, MacFayden BV, Palazzo F. History of laparoscopic surgery. Panminerva Med. 2000;42:87-90.

Tissue Handling: "Gently does it"

Vasundhara Oberoi

■ INTRODUCTION

If you want to achieve surgical results that are acceptable to excellent, remember that the results depend largely on the techniques of tissue handling. Tissue handling, tissue traction, crusting, moisture, the prevention of desiccation, hemostasis, the use of electric and chemical contact, dressing, and the closure pressure determine soft tissue results.

■ HEMOSTASIS

The prevention of excessive blood loss makes for a clear surgical field, stabilizes the patient's hemodynamics; prevents hematoma, hence reducing tension at the margins of the wound; allows tissue to settle easily; prevents the formation of dead space; and reduces the medium for bacterial proliferation and hence, infection.

Hemostasis can be achieved by (i) promoting natural hemostasis, sponging, and pressure dabbing; (ii) thermal coagulation using heat in the form of electrocautery patients should be earthed and freed to be clear of liquids, forming sumps; (iii) suture ligation using nonresorbable and pliant sutures, with secure and multiple knots (double throw); or (iv) using procoagulants such as thrombin analogs in spray or impregnated pledgets.

■ MAINTAINING MOISTURE IN TISSUE

During long procedures, you may periodically irrigate the wound with warm physiological (normal) saline solution.

■ DEAD SPACE MANAGEMENT

Dead space in a wound results from the separation of portions of the wound beneath the edges of the skin that have not been closely approximated, or from air or fluid trapped between the layers of tissue. This is especially true of the fatty layer, which tends to lack blood supply. Serum or blood may collect in these layers, providing an ideal medium for the growth of microorganisms that cause infection. You may elect to insert a drain or apply a pressure dressing postoperatively to eliminate dead space in the wound. Dead space is best managed by:

- Deep tissue suturing, such as marsupialization suturing, to approximate surfaces
- Pressure dressing or placing packing material for 12–18 hours, when the cavity walls are not collapsible
- The use of drains to empty collected fluids by gravity, capillary, or suction-aided drains.

■ DECONTAMINATION AND DEBRIDEMENT

Adequate debridement of all devitalized tissue and the removal of inflicted foreign materials are essential to healing, especially in traumatic wounds. The presence of fragments of dirt, metal, glass, etc. increases the probability of infection. You must look for and excise dead and dying or devitalized tissue, using atraumatic and sharp dissection. The same goes for foreign material. Mechanical abraders and pulsed lavage can be used to dislodge macro- and microscopic debris, and antibiotics can be added to the lavage fluids in cases of heavy contamination.

■ CHOICE OF CLOSURE MATERIAL

You must evaluate each case individually and accordingly, choose the closure material which will maximize the opportunity for healing and minimize the likelihood of infection. The proper closure material will allow you to approximate tissue with the minimum trauma possible, with enough precision to eliminate dead space. The surgeon's personal preference plays a big role in the choice of the closure material, but his decision is also influenced by the location of the wound, the arrangement of the tissue fibers and factors related to the patient.

The suture material must have high and uniform tensile strength. It should retain its strength throughout the crucial healing phase and its diameter should be uniform. The material should be such that the passage of the suture though the tissue is nontraumatic. Finally, it should not elicit a marked tissue response.

■ CELLULAR RESPONSE TO CLOSURE MATERIAL

Tissues react whenever foreign material, such as sutures, are implanted in them. This reaction ranges from minimal to moderate, depending on the type of material implanted. The reaction is more marked if complicated by infection, allergy, or trauma. Initially, the tissue deflects the passage of the surgeon's needle and suture. Once the sutures have been implanted, edema of the skin and subcutaneous tissues ensues. This can cause significant discomfort during recovery, as well as scarring secondary to ischemic necrosis. The surgeon must take these factors into consideration when placing tension on the closure material.

■ CLOSING TENSION

While enough tension must be applied to approximate tissue and eliminate dead space, the sutures must be loose enough to minimize excessive patient discomfort, ischemia, and tissue necrosis during healing.

■ POSTOPERATIVE DISTRACTION FORCES

The patient's postoperative activity can place undue stress on a healing incision. For example, there will be excessive tension on the abdominal fascia after a surgery if the patient strains to cough, vomit, void, or defecate. Tendons and the extremities may also be subjected to excessive tension during healing. You must make sure that the approximated wound is adequately immobilized to prevent suture disruption for a certain period of time.

■ IMMOBILIZATION

Adequate immobilization of the approximated wound, but not necessarily of the entire anatomical part, is mandatory after surgery for efficient healing and minimal scar formation.

■ SUGGESTED READING

1. Booth PW, Eppley B, Schmelzeisen R. Maxillofacial Trauma and Esthetic Facial Reconstruction - Elsevier eBook on VitalSource (Retail Access Card), 2nd Edition, 2012.
2. Eugene B, Kern MD, David A, Sherris MD. Mayo Clinic Basic Surgical Skills. Mayo Clinic Scientific Press; 1999.
3. Hupp JR, Ellis III E, Tucker MR. Contemporary Oral and Maxillofacial Surgery. Sixth Edition, Elsevier, 2014.
4. Mangram AJ, Horan TC, Pearson ML, Silver LC, Jarvis WR. Guideline for prevention of surgical site infection, 1999. Hospital Infection Control Practices Advisory Committee. Infect Control Hosp Epidemiol. 1999;20:250-78; quiz 279-80.

Surgeon and His Tools

13

Catheters and Cannulas

Ashish Dey

■ INTRODUCTION

The word "catheter" originates from the Latin "kathe," which means "to send down." Catheters are hollow, flexible plastic tubes that can be inserted into a body cavity, duct or vessel for diagnostic or therapeutic purposes. They can be simple or self-retaining. The latter are balloon catheters, e.g., Foley catheters. A urinary catheter drains urine from the bladder, while a vascular catheter is inserted into small vessels. Catheters allow for the drainage of fluids or the injection of fluids into a system. They may also be used to distend lumen or provide access to the surgical instrumentation.

A catheter consists of a hub, a body and an atraumatic "tip." Various polymers are used to make catheters. These are inert. The most commonly used polymers are silicone, polyvinyl chloride, polyethylene, Teflon, polyurethane, rubber or latex. Silicone catheters can be used for a month or more. The ideal characteristics of a catheter are strength and flexibility, depending on its use in various body systems, radiopacity, and low surface frictional resistance so that it can be guided over guide wire, as in the case of vascular catheters.

Size of catheter: The French scale or French gauge system is commonly used to measure the size of a catheter. The French size, most often abbreviated as Fr, measures the outer diameter of a catheter. It is thrice the millimeter. The diameter of a round catheter in millimeters can be determined by dividing the French size by 3, that is, diameter (mm) = Fr/3. For example, if the French size is 9, the diameter is 9/3 = 3 mm. An increasing French size corresponds to a larger external diameter. This is in contrast to the needle gauge, in which an increasing gauge corresponds to a needle of a smaller diameter. The English system, according to which the external diameter was E/2 + 1, is no longer in use.

The important guiding principle in choosing the catheter to be used is that the smallest size of catheter necessary to maintain adequate drainage is to be considered. Larger caliber catheters are chosen if debris or clots are expected to drain.

■ TYPES OF CATHETERS

Urinary Catheters

The urinary catheters used most commonly are Foley catheters. The Malecot catheter, a ureteral catheter, is no longer in use and ureteric catheters are now called *stents*. At the proximal end of the two-way Foley catheter are two openings, one of which is used to push water into the subterminal bulb and another terminal opening to be fitted with a reservoir bag. The other end is closed with a subterminal side opening that makes the insertion of the catheter atraumatic. The Foley catheter may be used for diagnostic or therapeutic purposes. As far as diagnosis is concerned, it is used to collect uncontaminated urine specimens, study the anatomy of the urinary tract and monitor the urine output. As for the therapeutic uses of Foley catheters, they are effective in acute urinary retention, chronic obstruction causing hydronephrosis and intermittent bladder decompression for neurogenic bladder. It is absolutely essential to use aseptic techniques during insertion.

A Foley catheter may also be three-way, i.e., with three channels. One is for balloon inflation, one for drainage and an extra one for irrigation. The external diameter of the latter is similar to that of the other two channels. The extra channel is used after prostate surgery for continued irrigation to prevent blood clots from causing obstruction. The ideal fluid for inflating the balloon is distilled water and not normal saline, which precipitates in hot water. Air would make the balloon float and cause irritation to the trigone, and may even make the balloon rupture easily. It is important to take good care of the catheter and bladder washes may be necessary if the catheter is retained for a long time.

In emergency situations, the Foley catheter can be used as a tube to deliver oxygen, a suction catheter and a tourniquet to prevent blood loss. It is also used to administer rectal enema, retract delicate structures during surgery and test anastomotic integrity after rectal surgery.

The size of Foley catheters varies from 8 to 24 Fr, but the most commonly used ones are 14 and 16 Fr. The sizes available and color code used in surgical practice are mentioned in **Table 1**.

Vascular Catheters

These may be Swan–Ganz catheters or vascular embolectomy catheters. They are open at both ends. They are either diagnostic catheters, used for angiographs, or guiding catheters, used for angioplasty. The latter are stiffer than diagnostic catheters as they carry balloon catheters, percutaneous transluminal coronary angioplasty (PTCA) wires and stent delivery systems. They may have end holes or side holes. The size of adult diagnostic angiographic catheters ranges from 5 to 7 Fr.

TABLE 1: Color code and size of Foley catheters.

Color code	Size	Balloon capacity	Length of catheters
Black	8 Fr	3 mL/cc	250 mm
Gray	10 Fr	3 mL/cc	250 mm
White	12 Fr	10 mL/cc	380 mm
Green	14 Fr	10 mL/cc	380 mm
Orange	16 Fr	20 mL/cc	380 mm
Red	18 Fr	20 mL/cc	380 mm
Yellow	20 Fr	20 mL/cc	380 mm
Purple	22 Fr	50 mL/cc	380 mm
Blue	24 Fr	50 mL/cc	380 mm

Gauge	Color code	External diameter (mm)	Length (mm)	Flow rate (mL/min)
14G	Orange	2.1	45	240
16G	Gray	1.8	45	180
18G	Green	1.3	32/45	90
20G	Pink	1.1	32	60
22G	Blue	0.9	25	36
24G	Yellow	0.7	19	20
26G	Violet	0.6	19	13

TABLE 2: Color code and size of cannulas.

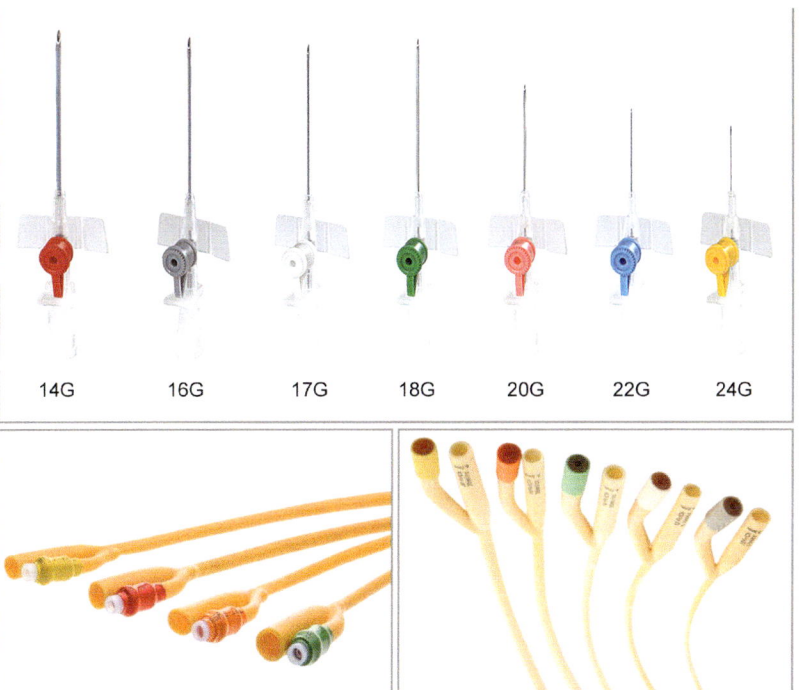

14G   16G   17G   18G   20G   22G   24G

Fig. 1: Color coding for various intravenous cannulas (above) and Foley catheters (below).

Depending on the type, catheters can be used for a variety of applications. Placing a catheter into a particular part of the body may allow for the drainage of a collection of fluid, as is the case with an abdominal abscess.

■ CANNULAS

A cannula is a tube that can be inserted into the body, often for the delivery or removal of fluid or for gathering data. A cannula usually surrounds the outer surface of a metallic hollow needle called "trocar." An example is an IV cannula. Its size mostly ranges from 14 to 24G (Gauze). Cannulas of different sizes have different color codes, as specified in **Table 2** and **Figure 1**. A venous cannula is inserted into a vein primarily for the administration of intravenous fluids, obtaining blood samples and administering medicines. An IV drip set is attached to the cannula. It has a three-way channel, polyvinyl chloride (PVC) tubing, a rubber tube and a Murphy's chamber. The Murphy's chamber has a filter and provides a window through which one can see and control the rate of infusion. An arterial cannula is inserted into an artery, mostly the radial artery, during major operations and in the intensive care unit to measure intra-arterial real-time blood pressure and to draw repeated arterial blood samples for gas analysis.

Intravenous Cannulas

Intravenous (IV) cannulas are another variety of catheters. Peripheral or central venous catheters are employed to administer intravenous fluids, medication or parenteral nutrition. Central venous catheters deliver drugs or fluids into a large vein or just inside the atrium. Various catheters make it possible to directly measure blood pressure in an artery or vein. A Swan–Ganz catheter is a special type of catheter that is placed into the pulmonary artery to measure pressures in the heart. Epidural catheters allow for the direct measurement of intracranial pressure, as also the administration of anesthetic medication into the epidural space, into the subarachnoid space or around a major nerve bundle, such as the brachial plexus.

■ CONCLUSION

Choosing the appropriate cannula and catheter size in the clinical setting is of utmost importance as delivery of the appropriate drugs and fluids at appropriate speed has a bearing on the prognosis, patient comfort and recovery.

Electrocautery—Arts and Principles: A Fundamental Concept

Deep Goel

■ INTRODUCTION

Bleeding has always been a nightmare for surgeons. Compression, either manual or using an instrument, and suturing were used to achieve hemostasis in ancient times. The use of heat for the treatment of wounds dates back to the Neolithic Age. Later, bleeding was controlled with hot irons. In the mid-eighteenth century, direct current (DC) was used for therapeutic purposes by way of heat being transferred from an instrument heated by the passage of an electric. Jacques-Arsène d'Arsonval, the French physicist, inventor and physiologist, was the first to report the use of alternating current (AC) in the clinical context in 1893. In 1907, Rivère, a student of d'Arsonval, demonstrated that if high-frequency AC was applied directly to the tissue without sparking, an electrosurgical process called "white coagulation" occurred. The first electrosurgical unit was introduced by Bovie in 1928. Since 1929, when AJ McLean described radiofrequency electrosurgery, or the effects of electric current on tissues, there have been considerable advancements in electrosurgery. It is now possible for the surgeons to cut or coagulate the target tissue by applying high-frequency electrical current to it, making for a virtually bloodless surgery. This method has become the greatest assistant for all surgeons.

In radiofrequency electrosurgery, electromagnetic energy is converted first to kinetic energy, then to thermal energy. Usually, a frequency of around 500 kHz is used, which is the same as the frequency of amplitude modification (AM) radio broadcasts **(Fig. 1)**. Hence, the use of the term radiofrequency (RF) electrosurgery.

Electrosurgery is different from electrocautery or diathermy. Electrosurgery refers to the passage of high-frequency AC through the tissue to produce the desired effect.

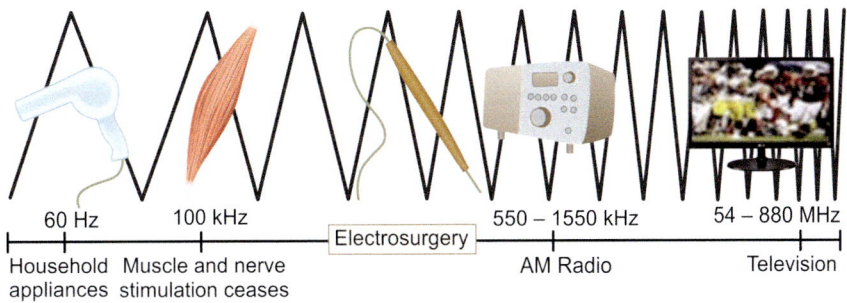

60 Hz	100 kHz	Electrosurgery	550 – 1550 kHz	54 – 880 MHz
Household appliances	Muscle and nerve stimulation ceases		AM Radio	Television

Fig. 1: Waveforms and the fields in which they are used.

In contrast, an electrical current is used to heat a surgical instrument and the heat is transferred to the tissue for the desired effects, in electrocautery. The term "surgical diathermy" is used as a synonym for electrosurgery, but in fact, diathermy means dielectric heating, produced by the rotation of molecular dipoles in a high-frequency electromagnetic field. Diathermy may be physical (ultrasound, short-wave and microwave diathermy) or surgical (electrocautery).

◼ ELECTROPHYSICAL PRINCIPLE

In an electrical circuit, current flows from a positive (active) electrode to a negative (return) electrode. Human tissues conduct current only when the circuit is complete. If the circuit is incomplete, the tissues get heated, and this is the core principle of electrosurgery. The amount of heat produced is directly proportional to the current density, tissue resistance and amount of time, and inversely, to the cross-sectional area of the active electrode, as described by Joule's law. So, a smaller electrode produces the desired effect in a small amount of time and the effect on the tissue depends on the rate of rise in temperature, which can be adjusted by electrosurgical generator settings. In electrocautery, the current passing through the hand instrument produces heat and the heat is transferred to the tissue for the desired effect.

◼ ELECTROSURGICAL UNITS

An electrosurgical unit (ESU) is an electrical circuit consisting of two electrodes (active and return), the patient, the electrosurgical generator, and the connecting wires. The two electrodes may be in either of two forms—(1) an active handpiece controlled by a foot pedal or hand-switch and a grounding plate (patient plate or dispersive pad) or (2) a combined hand instrument like forceps. The first one is called a monopolar system and the second is known as a bipolar system **(Fig. 2)**. It is important to remember that all radiofrequency electrosurgery is done with a bipolar instrument.

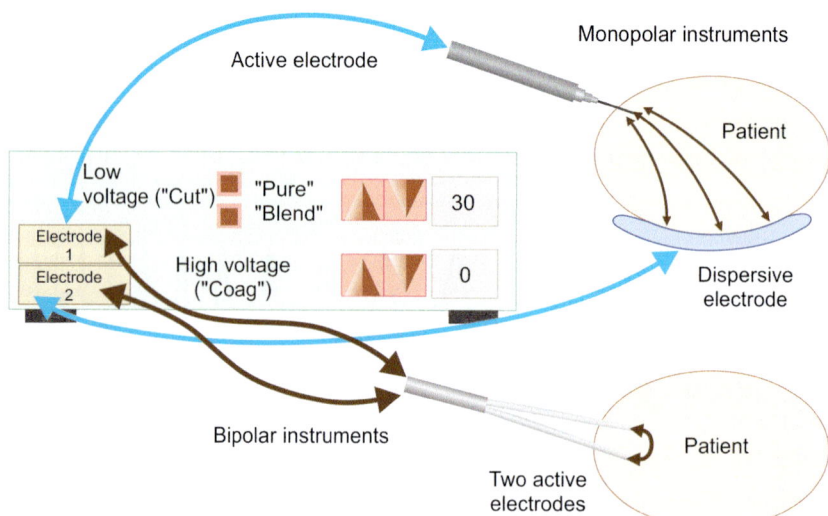

Fig. 2: Basic components of an electrosurgical unit with monopolar and bipolar instruments.

Electrosurgical generators are typically classified into (i) low power (50–100 W), for microsurgery, (ii) mid-range power (100–200 W), for most procedures, and (iii) high power (300–400 W), for coronary artery bypass graft (CABG) and transurethral resection of prostrate (TURP). Earlier, generators needed to be earthed, but now they are "isolated" and do not need to be earthed. Electrosurgical generators converts the low-frequency AC from a wall outlet into a radiofrequency output, typically from 300 to 500 kHz. At around 100 kHz, electric current can cause the "faradic effect" with possible muscular twitching, pain, even ventricular fibrillation and cardiac arrest causing harm to the patient. At or >5 MHz, current may leak, posing a threat to the patient and the surgeon. The range of output frequency (300 kHz to 5 MHz) is inherent to the device and varies according to the manufacturer and most importantly, cannot be adjusted according to the operating surgeon's choice. The generator power output is most often indicated in a digital display (in watts) on the face of the generator. Some machines may have a logarithmic scale from 1 (lowest) to 10 (highest), making the output interpretation difficult.

◼ ELECTRODE CONFIGURATION (CIRCUIT TOPOLOGY)

As mentioned earlier, an electrosurgical unit may be monopolar or bipolar. In the monopolar system, current flows from the generator through the active electrode into the target tissue, through the patient, the dispersive pad or patient plate (return electrode) and then returns to the generator **(Fig. 3A)**. If the patient plate (earlier known as indifferent plate) is properly placed, the desired effect will be only at the active electrode, not at the patient plate. This is of immense importance with regard to patient safety.

In contrast to monopolar settings, bipolar electrosurgery uses an active and a return electrode that are a small distant apart **(Fig. 3B)**. This allows the current to pass through the target tissue and return to the instrument via the return electrode, doing away with the need for a dispersive pad on the patient. The estimated depth of penetration in this case is 0.5–1 mm, compared with 3–5 mm for monopolar systems. The maximal lateral thermal spread is 5 mm. As the two electrodes are in close proximity, lower voltages are used. However, the bipolar system is not necessarily safe, as capacitive coupling can also cause injury.

◼ DISPERSIVE PAD (PATIENT PLATE)

The dispersive pad should (i) be near the site of the active electrode to decrease resistance from other tissues, (ii) have conductive gel to decrease skin resistance, and (iii) remain in complete contact all the time. If the dispersive pad does not make sufficient contact with the patient's skin, alternative site burn can occur. It should be placed on clean, dry skin over a large muscle mass, avoiding bony areas and scar tissue. The primary purpose of the dispersive pad is to provide a grounding path from the patient back to the generator and ensure an area of low current density. If this point is compromised, the circuit will then be completed through other grounded contact points such as the metal table touching the patient, electrocardiogram (ECG) leads, towel clips, and intravenous fluid stands.

It must be remembered that the amount of energy delivered to the active electrode is the same as that delivered to the patient plate, but the current density at the two sites is very

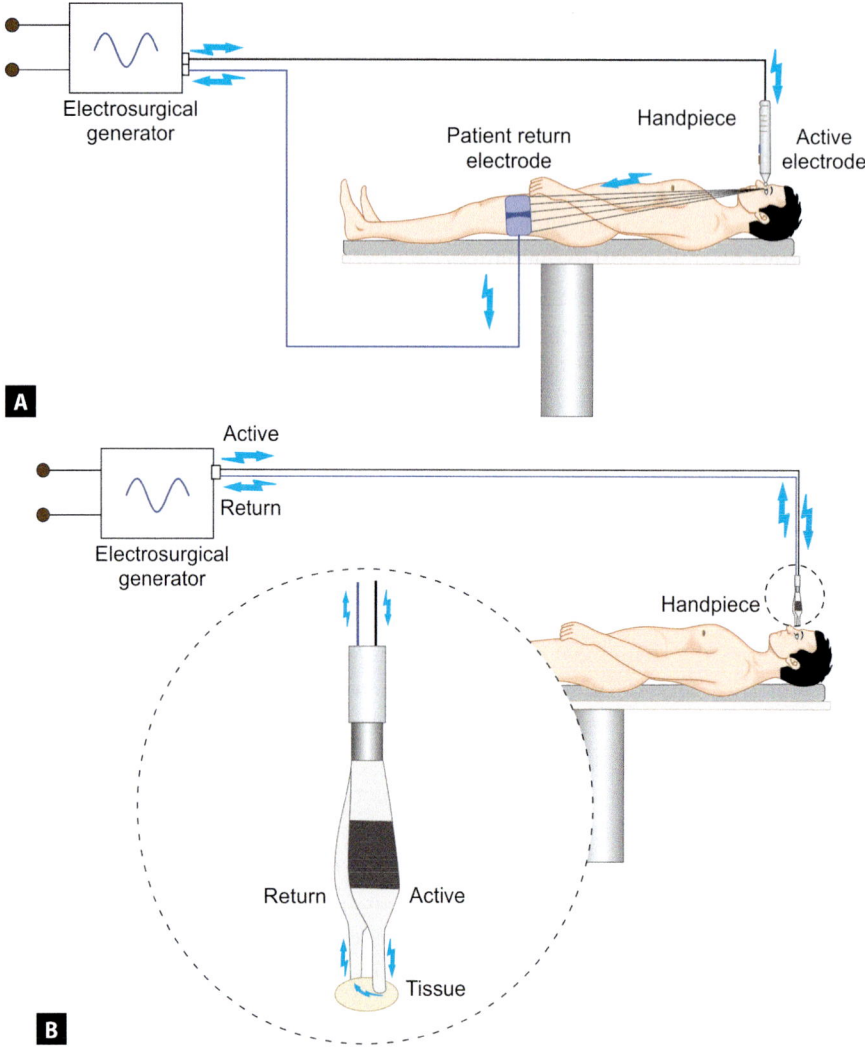

Figs. 3A and B: (A) Monopolar system and (B) Bipolar system.

different because the active end is much smaller than the patient plate. If the patient plate is small or inappropriately placed, it will cause burns. Burn injuries can be prevented by using a dual-pad and a return electrode monitoring (REM) circuit. The REM circuit detects changes in surface/resistance and shuts off the unit automatically. It is available in modern electrosurgical units.

■ MODES AND WAVEFORMS

The AC waveform is modulated in accordance with the mode of electrosurgery. There are three types—(1) cutting current (continuous, unmodulated, and undampened), (2) blended current (different percentage duty cycle), and (3) coagulation current (interrupted, modulated, and

TABLE 1: Comparison between the cut and coagulation modes.

Mode	Cut	Coagulation
Color coding	Yellow	Blue
Current flow	High current energy, relatively low voltage	High voltage, short, and interrupted current bursts with current-free intervals
Waveform	Continuous, unmodulated, and undampened	Dampened wave with a 6% duty cycle in "off" and "on" mode (i.e., 6% of the time "on" and 94% "off")
Rise of temperature	Quick increase	Slow rise
Tissue effects	Vaporization of tissue water and fragmentation	Thermal protein denaturing (at 70–80°C "white coagulation") and with time desiccation
Depth of effect	Less deep	Deeper tissue injury
Submodes	Pure cut blend	Desiccate fulgurate Spray

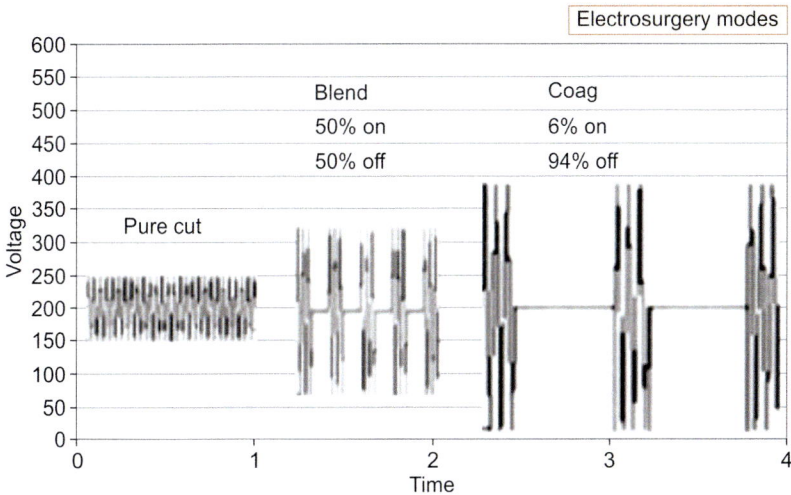

Fig. 4: "On" and "off" duty cycles in different modes.

dampened). The last is used to attain hemostasis, occlude lumen-containing structures or destroy a large volume of tissue such as soft tissue neoplasms. **Table 1** compares the two basic modes.

In modern electrosurgical generators, these modes have different preset submodes **(Table 1)**. The current has a 100% "on" duty cycle, i.e., it is always "on" in the pure cut (vaporization) mode **(Fig. 4)**. A quick rise in temperature to 100°C or beyond, causes intracellular water to boil, forming steam and results in explosive vaporization of the cell. During the cooling periods, cell wall explosion and vaporization are accompanied by the slow dehydration of cellular fluid and protein. The pure cut effect is produced by a pointed

TABLE 2: Comparison between the cut and coagulation modes.

Purpose	Recommended mode	Typical electrode
Incising tissue	Pure cut	Blade type
Excising tissue	Pure cut	Loop type
Desiccation	Blend (cut)	Blade, blunt needle or ball type
Fulguration	Coagulation	Blunt needle (pinpoint) or ball type (cone spray)

or thin loop-shaped electrode held close to, but not in contact with, the tissue. The current concentrating at the tip then arcs to the tissue resulting in a rapid rise in temperature causing vaporization. So, in short, cutting needs a short cooling time or low crest factor (generator's ability to coagulate without cutting) and slightly loose contact.

The blend mode is a variation of the cutting mode with a higher duty cycle (usually 12–80% "on") than in the pure coagulation mode **(Fig. 4)**. It is a blend of surgical effects or blended outputs. The blend effect by variations of dampened currents based on the surgeon's choice and desired effect. On this basis, blend may have blend 1 or 2 or 3 modes according to the percentage of duty cycle. A quick rise in temperature to $90°C$ (but not $100°C$) dehydrates the cells, while preserving their architecture, but if longer cooling time than pure cut is available, desiccation will occur. Desiccation can be achieved in both the cut and coagulation modes. Even a bipolar electrode with both blades in contact can desiccate tissue when a cutting current is used. Desiccation needs a high crest factor and close contact. When the temperature rises to $200°C$ or more, carbonization (fulguration or black coagulation) occurs. Sweeping movement of the active electrode, held a few millimeters away from the tissue, causes intermittent high-voltage sparks across the gap, resulting in broad and superficial coagulation. This mode of coagulation is known as spray coagulation. Sweeping avoids charring of tissue. The most common indication for using this mode is an oozing capillary bed over a wide area. Fulguration needs a high peak voltage and very loose contact. It can be achieved in both monopolar and bipolar configurations. Most modern bipolar units achieve excellent desiccation and coagulation at low settings (15–20 W). However, bipolar electrodes cannot be used effectively for a cutting effect as it is difficult for the two electrodes to be oriented in such a way as to allow efficient vaporization to occur. **Table 2** summarizes the uses of the different modes.

■ ELECTROSURGICAL INJURY

Electrothermal injuries are quite common and most importantly, they are preventable. These injuries are of major concern from the patient's perspective. They may result from:

- The dispersive electrode due to application site issues and partial detachment (already discussed earlier)
- Current diversion due to insulation failure, direct coupling, capacitive coupling, alternate site injuries
- The active electrode due to inadvertent activation or direct trauma.

Direct coupling occurs due to unintended contact with a noninsulated instrument (e.g., laparoscope, metal grasper forceps) within the abdomen. Electric current then flows from the active electrode into the secondary conductor and energizes it. Capacitive coupling occurs when electric current is transferred from one conductor (the active electrode), through intact insulation, to adjacent conductive materials (e.g., bowel) without direct contact. It is classically seen in minimally invasive surgery. It occurs when a nonconductive (plastic) locking anchor of a hybrid conductive (metal) sleeve insulates the abdominal wall from the current and the current bleeds off a metal sleeve or laparoscope into the viscera. This may result in thermal necrosis and a delayed fecal fistula. Single-port laparoscopic surgery is associated with this type of injury. Current diversion may occur when elements of the circuit interface with any conductive structure, resulting in alternate site injury. This phenomenon is much less common in the case of modern machines, as they automatically shut down when they detect a reduced current flow because of an AC pathway. A common issue specific to laparoscopic surgery is complications from unrecognized energy transfer, called stray current. It may occur either within or outside the operational field of view.

Out of the two electrosurgical modalities, monopolar electrosurgery causes far greater thermal damage. Studies have shown that the bipolar device has the least amount of thermal spread among the various energy-based devices and provides safe sealing and coagulation quality that are similar to other energy-based devices. Some injuries (such as the mushroom effect and adherence to target tissue) are specific to the bipolar modality. In bipolar instruments, as energy is delivered from both jaws to a target vessel from the outside, the superficial tissues became desiccated and visibly change color even before the core tissues reach denaturation states sufficient for hemostasis. Also, unabated application of energy to a target vessel increases its electrical resistance (impedance) due to the loss of water (desiccation) and results in the preferential flow of current through less resistive, surrounding tissues. This mushroom effect extends the risk of collateral damage beyond the lateral thermal spread, making it necessary for surgeons to estimate the correct time for stopping energy delivery. Occasionally, a bipolar device may become "stuck" or adhere to the target tissue. Care must be taken to minimize traumatic detachment, and the use of mechanical force is discouraged as this may cause disruption of the newly created vessel seal. Reactivation of the bipolar device under irrigation will create steam bubbles that may help to dislodge the tissue. An alternative is to reactivate the bipolar device with minimal jaw apposition (to "reheat" the protein bonds at the tissue-device interface). The tunnel effect is an injury specific to the monopolar modality. There are some surgeons who are fond of doing circumcisions using monopolar diathermy and sometimes they are surprised to find the entire piece turn black and fall-off. The basic point is that while using electrocautery on any structure, you must be sure that the base of the structure is wider than the part that is being cauterized. If it is a tubular structure that is narrower in the middle than on top, the electrical circuits will cross, the currents will also cross making a crisscross. This is what is called the *tunnel effect*. The maximum heat is generated at the base. That is why while cauterizing something delicate, you should take care not to lift it into the air so that there is enough of a common base.

Electrothermal injuries may not be detected at the time of the operation or hemostasis, but later they may cause problems like stricture (commonly common bile duct injuries in laparoscopic cholecystectomy) or delayed perforation by ischemia due to the lateral spread of current or heat. Generally speaking, symptoms of delayed bowel perforation following electrothermal injury are usually seen 4–10 days after the procedure.

The operating team too faces certain occupational hazards associated with electrocautery. Surgical gloves can pass radiofrequency current by hydration (low resistance conduction), capacitive coupling (induced charge from the hemostat to the sweating conductive skin of the surgeon), and high-voltage dielectric breakdown (e.g., holes in gloves). Hence, surgeons should consider replacing their gloves during long procedures that expose the gloves to large amounts of blood or fluid. Glove resistance decreases with time and exposure to saline (e.g., sweat). The risk of a capacitive coupling injury through surgical gloves is inversely proportional to the glove's thickness and increases with higher voltage and longer contact time. Electrocautery plumes contain ultrafine particles and volatile chemical and biological substances, of which a number are teratogenic or carcinogenic.

Prevention of Electrosurgical Injuries

Most electrothermal injuries can be prevented if the operating team is well-coordinated and cautious. Always ensure that all connections to the generator are made before switching it on. You must have a thorough understanding of the biophysical principles of electrocautery.

- When the generator output does not produce the desired effects, check the patient plate and its connection and check the circuit integrity, instead of increasing the power output. Always respect the "alarm" of the generator. It will get silenced automatically if the circuit is complete.
- Always check the patient plate if the patient is moved during surgery and place the plate as close to the operative site as possible.
- Make sure that the diathermy cord is free of kinks, knots and bends, which could damage the cord or cause leakage, current accumulation and overheating of the insulation.
- Do not perform an electrosurgical procedure in the presence of gastrointestinal gases and in an oxygen-rich environment. Gastrointestinal gases contain hydrogen and methane, which are highly flammable. Fire and patient injuries may occur.
- Do not activate the active electrode in the presence of flammable agents (e.g. antimicrobial skin prep or hand antisepsis agents, tinctures, defatting agents, petroleum-based lubricants, phenol, aerosol adhesives, uncured methyl methacrylate) until the agents are dry and vapors have dissipated.
- Be cautious about the coagulation mode as it is intermittent, which necessitates a higher voltage than that needed to achieve comparable power in the cutting current mode, and predisposes to the potential arcing to nontarget tissue.
- Avoid hybrid trocar sleeves in laparoscopic surgery.
- Take care to ensure that the tissue to be cauterized is not to be too thick. The greater the tissue thickness between the jaws of an instrument, the greater is the amount (Joules) of energy that is required for complete coagulation and desiccation. So, thicker pedicles result in greater lateral extension of electrosurgical thermal injury, a factor that may be enhanced in the case of monopolar instruments.
- At the end of a procedure, undo all the connections and then switch off the machine. Never do it in the reverse order.

- Be extra cautious if the patient has a pacemaker because the circuit of the electrocautery unit can interfere with the electromagnetic circuit of the pacemaker and cause serious problems such as arrhythmias, or even cause the pacemaker to stop working. It is preferable not to use electrocautery in such cases. Other types of energy sources such as the harmonic scalpel are now available. If you must use electrocautery, opt for the bipolar system. Place the plate far away from the pacemaker site and use the electric supply in short bursts. Preferably, carry out the procedure in the presence of a cardiologist.

■ TREATMENT OF BURNS

Always check the patient plate site and other vulnerable sites for electrosurgical burns when the operation is over. Generally, these are full-thickness burns. So, they require full-thickness excision, apart from the application of dressings of nanocrystalline silver compounds. Always inform the hospital administration. You may be aware that in western countries, there are special electromagnetic teams to deal with such problems because they form a very big medico-legal issue. So, you must inform the hospital administration that a cautery burn has been caused in a particular theater in a particular patient and under a particular surgeon. You must definitely inform the patient about the burn and about the treatment of the burn.

To conclude, before using electrocautery you must understand the machine and the biophysical principles on which it works to ensure the safety of the patient and of the surgical team. Any preventable unintentional harm to the patient is considered medical negligence under the law.

■ SUGGESTED READING

1. Box GN, Lee HJ, Abraham JB, Deane LA, Elchico ER, Abdelshehid CA, et al. Comparative study of in vivo lymphatic sealing capability of the porcine thoracic duct using laparoscopic dissection devices. J Urol. 2009;181(1):387-91.
2. Brunt ML. Fundamentals of Electrosurgery Part II: Thermal Injury Mechanisms and Prevention. In: Feldman L, Fuchshuber P, Jones D (Eds). The SAGES Manual on the Fundamental Use of Surgical Energy (FUSE). New York, NY: Springer; 2012.
3. Bussiere RL. Principles of electrosurgery. Edmonds (WA): Tektran Incorporated; 1997.
4. Cordero I. Electrosurgical units – how they work and how to use them safely. Community Eye Health. 2015;28(89):15-6.
5. Cushing H, Bovie W. Electrosurgery as an aid to the removal of intracranial tumors. Surg Gynecol Obstet. 1928;47(6):751-84.
6. Jones CM, Pierre KB, Nicoud IB, Stain SC, Melvin 3rd WV. Electrosurgery. Curr Surg. 2006;63(6):458-63.
7. Kelly HA, Ward GE. Electrosurgery. Philadelphia: WB Saunders; 1932.
8. Martin DC, Soderstrom RM, Hulka JF, et al. Electrosurgery safety. Am Assoc Gynecol Laparosc Tech Bull. 1995;1:1-7.
9. Massarweh NN, Cosgriff N, Slakey DP. Electrosurgery: History, principles, and current and future uses. J Am Coll Surg. 2006; 202(3):520-30.
10. Matthews B, Nalysnyk L, Estok R, Fahrbach K, Banel D, Linz H, et al. Ultrasonic and nonultrasonic instrumentation: A systematic review and meta-analysis. Arch Surg. 2008; 143(6):592-600.
11. McLean A. The Bovie electrosurgical current generator: Some underlying principles and results. Arch Surg. 1929;18:1863-73.

12. Moak E. Electrosurgical unit safety. The role of the perioperative nurse. AORN J. 1991;53(3):744-6,748-9,752.
13. Munro MG. Energy sources for operative laparoscopy. In: Gomel V, Taylor PJ (Eds). Diagnostic and Operative Gynecologic Laparoscopy. St Louis: Mosby; 1995. pp. 26-56.
14. Munro MG. In: Feldman L, Fuchshuber P, Jones D (Eds). Fundamentals of Electrosurgery Part I: Principles of Radiofrequency Energy for Surgery. The SAGES Manual on the Fundamental Use of Surgical Energy (FUSE). New York: Springer; 2012.
15. Odell RC. Electrosurgery: Biophysics, safety and efficacy. In: Mann WJ, Stovall TG (Eds). Mann/Stovall Gynecologic Surgery. New York: Churchill Livingstone; 1996. pp. 55-67.
16. Odell RC. Electrosurgery: Principles and safety issues. Clin Obstet Gynecol. 1995; 38(3):610-21.
17. Odell RC. Laparoscopic electrosurgery. In: Hunter JG, Sackier JM (Eds). Minimally Invasive Surgery. New York: McGraw-Hill; 1993. p. 33.
18. Park CW, Portenier DD. Bipolar electrosurgical devices. In: Feldman L, Fuchshuber P, Jones D (Eds). The SAGES Manual on the Fundamental Use of Surgical Energy (FUSE). New York, NY: Springer; 2012.
19. Peterson HB, Ory HW, Greenspan JR, Tyler CW Jr. Deaths associated with laparoscopic sterilization by unipolar electrocoagulating devices, 1978 and 1979. Am J Obstet Gynecol. 1981;139(2):141-3.
20. Phipps JH. Understanding electrosurgery: Safety and efficiency. In: Lower A, Sutton C, Grudzinskas G (Eds). Introduction to Gynecological Endoscopy. Oxford, UK: Iris Medical Media; 1996. pp. 39-56.
21. Recommended Practices for Electrosurgery. In: Blanchard B, Burlingame B (Eds). Perioperative Standards and Recommended Practices. Denver, CO: Association of perioperative Registered Nurses, Inc; 2012. pp. 99-118.
22. Sutton PA, Awad S, Perkins AC, Lobo DN. Comparison of lateral thermal spread using monopolar and bipolar diathermy, the Harmonic Scalpel and the Ligasure. Br J Surg. 2010;97(3):428-33.
23. Taheri A, Mansoori P, Sandoval LF, Feldman SR, Pearce D, Williford PM. Electrosurgery: Part I. Basics and principles. J Am Acad Dermatol. 2014;70(4):591.e1-591.e14.
24. Tucker RD, Ferguson S. Do surgical gloves protect staff during electrosurgical procedures? Surgery. 1991;110(5):892-5.
25. Tucker RD, Schmitt OH, Sievert CE, Silvis SE. Demodulated low frequency currents from electrosurgical procedures. Surg Gynecol Obstet. 1984;159(1):39-43.
26. Voyles CR, Tucker RD. Education and engineering solutions for potential problems with laparoscopic monopolar electrosurgery. Am J Surg. 1992;164(1):57-62.
27. Wang K, Advincula AP. "Current thoughts" in electrosurgery. Int J Gynecol Obstet. 2007;97(3):245-50.
28. Wu MP, Chen WI, Chou CY, et al. Electrosurgical injury in laparoscopy. Show Chwan Med J. 2000:2:9-15.
29. Wu MP, Ou CS, Chen SL, Yen EY, Rowbotham R. Complications and recommended practices for electrosurgery in laparoscopy. Am J Surg. 2000;179(1):67-73.

15

Hypodermic Needles— Intramuscular and Intravenous

Harsha Jauhari

■ INTRODUCTION

This part is a bit historical. When I was a student, we had a professor of medicine and health who was very well known. He asked us who or what was a doctor. We all came up with our own answers, but he was not satisfied. Then he told us what he thought and I found it very relevant. I remember it even now after all these long years. He said a doctor is a person who, when he is woken up in the middle of the night, when everybody has tried and failed, comes to the hospital and puts a drip or puts in a nasogastric tube or the lumbar puncture or puts in a catheter in the first attempt after everybody else has tried and failed. And the beauty of it is that nobody has ever seen him doing it routinely. What this implies is that in your training period, you should do so many of these procedures that they become your second nature and you can do them blindly. However, you must learn the safe, scientific and successful way of doing these procedures. There are ways which are not so good.

Let us begin with a brief history of intramuscular (IM) and intravenous (IV) needles. In 1665, Sir Christopher Wren administered the first intravenous injection into a dog, and he was successful. Francis Boyle followed him. Now, Christopher Wren was the person who made St Paul's cathedral, so you can imagine the range of the man's talent. In 1853, almost 200 years later, the hypodermic syringe and needle were invented by Alexander Wood at Edinburgh. Charles Gabriel Pravaz invented the glass syringe (Gabriel syringe) independently at around the same time. In 1906, the first syringe of metal and glass was introduced in Berlin, and the Luer lock followed soon.

You must realize how lucky you are to have disposable syringes and needles, single use, are part and parcel of your day's work, you require to think twice. When we were interns, we had to use these horrible Cheatle forceps to pick up needles from boilers. We would try to ensure that nobody was looking, put up needle against the tip to see if there was a hook and then said this needle is good. We did not have cannulas. We used thick plastic tubes that came in little boxes and fed them onto certain needles. Glass syringes have a particular slot. If you don't get it right, they get jammed. As a result, every ward would have piles of jammed and discarded syringes. So, count yourself lucky that you have single-use syringes and needles.

■ GAUGE OF A NEEDLE

There are three parts to a needle. There is the barrel, the front part of it, there is a shaft and there is the hub which connects to a syringe. Now, in the business of gauge of a needle is

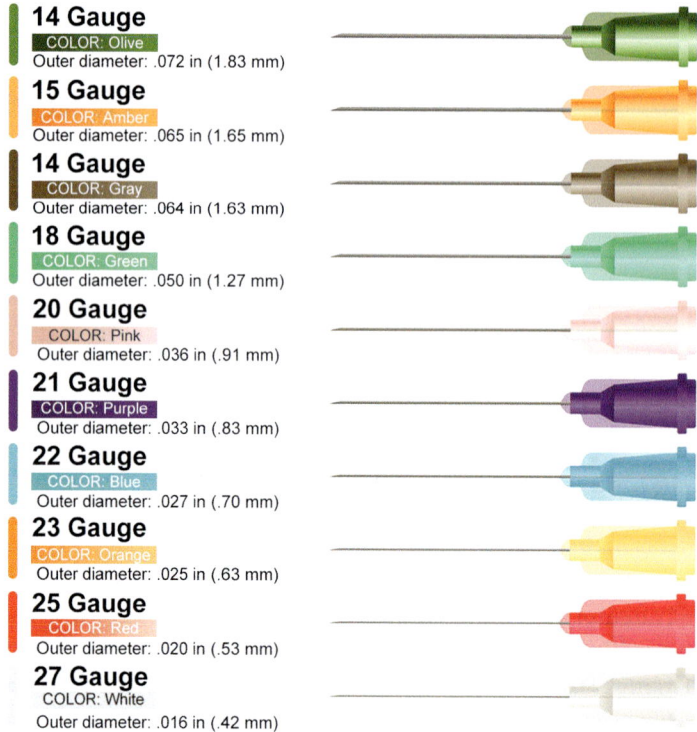

14 Gauge
COLOR: Olive
Outer diameter: .072 in (1.83 mm)

15 Gauge
COLOR: Amber
Outer diameter: .065 in (1.65 mm)

14 Gauge
COLOR: Gray
Outer diameter: .064 in (1.63 mm)

18 Gauge
COLOR: Green
Outer diameter: .050 in (1.27 mm)

20 Gauge
COLOR: Pink
Outer diameter: .036 in (.91 mm)

21 Gauge
COLOR: Purple
Outer diameter: .033 in (.83 mm)

22 Gauge
COLOR: Blue
Outer diameter: .027 in (.70 mm)

23 Gauge
COLOR: Orange
Outer diameter: .025 in (.63 mm)

25 Gauge
COLOR: Red
Outer diameter: .020 in (.53 mm)

27 Gauge
COLOR: White
Outer diameter: .016 in (.42 mm)

Fig. 1: Chart size of needle gauges for injections.

not the French gauge. The French gauge has to do with the diameter of a tube **(Fig. 1)**. It was originally based on the number of needles that fit into a square inch. That is why the higher the gauge number, the smaller is the size of the needle. If the size is 20, it means that 20 needles will fit into a square centimeter. However, now we use the internal diameter for gauge measurement and it ranges from 26G, which is 13 mm long and an internal diameter as you can see is of 0.45. The flow rate of approximately 13 mL/min to a 14G which is the largest needle used in the world by large and with an internal diameter of 2 mm and flow rate of 270 mL/min, that is a huge amount to be administered on the patient.

■ PARTS OF A NEEDLE

A needle has three parts. The front part is the bevel. Then there is the shaft and then the hub, which connects to the syringe. The hub of the needle may have a lock. The unlocked ones are the common in aspiration and injections. The locked ones with the Luer lock, etc., are for injections and aspirations or pick up fluids. The hub may be attached to a plastic syringe or a glass syringe. Glass syringes have mostly been superseded by plastic ones. They are phenol or formaldehyde some of the thicker solutions. Essentially, plastic syringes are now in and most of the solutions are being used by injections are aqueous or very thin oily. Oil based solutions tend to adsorb not absorb, they tend to adsorb in long glass solutions. Which is why for these phenol, formaldehyde you usually use glass syringes, but they have lastly now gone out of fashion.

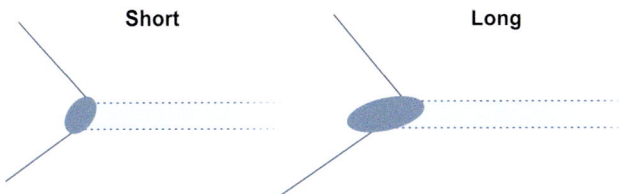

Fig. 2: Short and long bevels in Hypodermic needles.

Now, we consider the shaft. Never insert it fully. Roughly one-third of the needle should be out because if it breaks, you need enough length to hold and pull it out. It is no fun for a surgeon to try to take out a broken shaft from a joints or the deltoid muscle. Here is an interesting tip. Needles that are stored in a refrigerator tend to hurt less. This is probably because local cooling reduces pain.

Lastly, the bevel. It may be short or long **(Fig. 2)**. Obviously, a short bevel is as close to the internal diameter as possible. The long bevel, on the other hand, has a much larger area. A short bevel tends to damage more tissue where it goes in. A long bevel tends to separate the tissues, so it causes less damage. A short bevel is more useful at lesser depths. A long bevel delivers more over a wider area whereas, a short bevel delivers in front. It is important to know about this because if you have a needle half way into the vein and it has a long bevel. You will still get some blood and when you start injecting, you get extravasation. So, you should make sure that the bevel runs to the end. It is also of importance to remember the direction of the bevel in lumbar punctures (LP) and epidurals. If the patient is lying down, you do LP with the bevel up. The ligament fibers are parallel. You split the fibers, go in and turn it and nothing happens. But if the patient is sitting up and you still keep the bevel up and go straight in, you will tear the fibers the vein get you leaks. This is how infections occur. When it heals with fibrosis and scarring, the area will remain so tender that for the rest of the patient's life, he/she will jump with pain anytime someone touches it, and not remember you kindly or have nice things to say about you. Small things makes all the differences. The importance of the direction of the bevel.

■ INTRAMUSCULAR INJECTIONS

These are all very simple, the learner must remember a few basic things. Take the shortest route in; do not try to make funny designs **(Fig. 3)**. Go straight in. Pinch the skin and muscles when the patient has adequate subcutaneous fat or a taut skin. You have to stretch the skin or pinch it up. Always check for entering into a blood vessel by aspiration, in intramuscular injections. There are two good sites for IM injections—(1) the upper outer quadrants of the buttocks for deep IM and (2) the belly of the triceps, not the lateral head. The deltoid is not a good muscle to use as it is not an ovoid muscle. It is a flat muscle inserting as a "V." It is prone to going into the bone or hitting the blood vessels and nerves. In the deltopectoral groove, you may hit the cephalic vein. There are other sites that may be used, such as the lateral border of the thigh, but these are not commonly used.

All to do with transit through skin

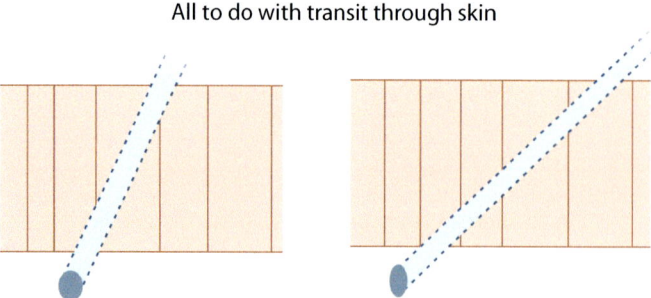

Fig. 3: Minimizing the pain.

Principles of Pain in Intramuscular Injection

Remember the following point:

- Wipe the area with a spirit swab and let it dry. You do not want to drive spirit into the wound.
- Make the shortest direct entry.
- If the patient is on anticoagulants or is a long-term user of aspirin, try to avoid intramuscular injections because they may cause hematomas.
- Do not inject >2.5 cc per injection site.
- Gently massage the area after withdrawal to allow the fluid to spread. Remember that you are not trying to ease the pain or make the area ischemic, you are only trying to spread the fluid.

■ INTRAVENOUS INJECTIONS

The veins that are commonly used are the basilic vein and the cephalic vein at the cubital fossa, the median cephalic vein at the dorsum of the hand, the wrist vein at the snuffbox, and the long saphenous vein at the ankle (although this is not a good choice for the long-term). The femoral, jugular and subclavian veins may be used in special situations or emergencies or when a large amount of fluid needs to be delivered in a short period of time, for dialysis, for example.

Principles of Pain in Intravenous Injection

Remember the following points:

- Do not hurry, not even in an emergency.
- Choose your vein carefully.
- Use a tourniquet cuff. If necessary, use a blood pressure (BP) monitor cuff. Inflate between diastolic or systolic and come back after two or three minutes. The veins will be distended. If you inflate the cuff above the systolic pressure, the vein will not become prominent for obvious reasons.
- Enter the skin as directly as possible. If it is a very big bulging vein, enter at a distance away from the vein, skin separately, vein separately.

- Take the sample with the cuff off or on, depending on what you require. There are times when you require to take off the cuff, for example, if you want to check calcium and potassium. In these cases, you will get wrong values if you have the cuff on.
- Inject fluids with the cuff off.
- If you are placing a cannula, fix it adequately.
- The elbow is a poor site for long-term infusion because it is very uncomfortable.
- Check regularly for inflammation thrombosis.

Some nurses do not cause pain when injecting. Do they do something different? Yes. The nerve fibers go up vertically. When you take the shortest route in, you damage only a few of them. When you make an acute angle, on the other hand, you tearing them. You may go through many nerve endings between the point of entry and the point of exit of an IV. This is what causes pain. The greater the distance between the points of entry and exit, the greater is the damage to free nerve endings. When you are withdrawing, remember that blood leaks from the vein and then from the skin. So, apply pressure on the puncture site and on the vein. You are trying to stop the bleeding from the puncture site, not inside.

This reminds me of an incident that occurred when I was an intern. I saw a senior approach a little child with a plastic syringe full of something with a peculiar smell (it was formaldehyde). The syringe had a size 14 needle and 10 cc of the fluid. I asked him where he was going. He said he was going to give the child an injection, but the child would just not shut up. I asked him where he planned to inject the fluid and he said, "in the buttock." I asked, "all of this?" He said, "Yes." I asked, "all in one place?" He said, "Yes." He was unsuccessful because the needle was too large for the child, the syringe was wrong for the drug and the needle size was wrong for the syringe. Also formaldehyde was wrong for the child, apart from the dose being wrong. Lastly, injecting 10 cc of the drug on one buttock of a small child is completely unacceptable.

So, in summary, giving injections we should take utmost care.

Needles—Solid Needles

Harsha Jauhari

■ INTRODUCTION

All surgical wounds require closure that is done with sutures on swaged needles in one or many layers. The attributes of each needle type is as important as the suture itself. One should correctly choose them according to the prevailing clinical situations and the surgical wound for optimal results. We will discuss when and where a particular needle needs to be used and why.

■ OLIVE-ENDED BLUNT NEEDLE

This is a fairly large needle that you use for the liver. You rarely use a needle holder with it because when you use a needle holder there is a loss of transmission of sensation. You virtually put it in with your hand as you keep feeling for the biliary radicle. Because when you use a needle holder there is a loss of transmission of sensation. So, when you have an olive-ended one, you gently tease it through, so all the rubbish gets separated and you move between the radicles to avoid causing any damage. You cannot use the taper cut on the liver. Another organ with very high vascularity is the kidney, where you can hit a blood vessel at any point. So, you try to take the simplest route when you go in. You cannot use a blunt needle because it will cause a lot of damage. The kidney will split, but the liver will not because the radicles will be held together and the soft tissue will be separated. If you use a blunt needle on the kidney, there will be a massive rupture. So, you cannot do that. Another place you do not want bleeding when can you use a reverse needle. The needle has got a thread. When can we use it backward? See what happens is, if you are stuck somewhere without a liver needle and you have to deal with massive bleeding? Then you take a large needle, hold it backward and go in the reverse direction. So you have doubled the back of the needle with the thread, and the thread serves like an olive-end. You can use it in the bulky mesentery during RA. If you use a sharp needle you will risk hitting a blood vessel and causing hematoma, so use the needle in reverse. You will feel some resistance only on the leaf of the peritoneum. The fat will separate, but you will never damage a blood vessel. The blood vessel will move away. This is a trick that you can use if you are ever in trouble. The reverse side of the needle will go through the peritoneum with a bit of resistance. All the other tissues will separate, come back the other side and you can tie it. For left-handed surgeons it should be practiced similarly.

■ SPATULA NEEDLE

This is used for ophthalmic surgery or microsurgery. It is flat so that you cause the minimum trauma to the tissue you are handling. You have to keep seeing the needle while passing it through the sclera. It remains flat. It does not fall sclera while passing through and as well as the tip and as a cutting edge so the tip passes. Again, you tell me two sides, cutting edge on the inner side and cutting edge on the outside.

The strong part of the suture is your needle not your suture. The more you keep clipping and clamping that, what is going to happen is, it is going to snap, especially the smaller ones. So good surgery involves not touching this at all. Sutures may be made of natural fibers or synthetic fibers. They may be braided or nonbraided. The braided ones have no memory, so it is easy to open them out. The monofilaments retain memory, so you have to break that.

■ THE RIGHT WAY TO HOLD THE NEEDLE

You have to work with the tip. If you are right-handed, go from the right to the left. If your assistant is right-handed, he will follow with the left hand, so that he can use his right hand to do something more meaningful, such as retracting or helping or supporting. Go from the right to the left, and the next bite will automatically suggest itself. If you are particular that you want to go from the left to the right, it is sometimes a good idea that you follow it yourself. There will be situations where you will use this reverse technique, so this is a skill you should all develop. It is a very, very sensible way of doing it when you are operating away from you.

If you are doing anastomosis of the bowel or a lumen or a vessel, do not think of it as joining two straight lines. You are joining two circles. They may be lying differently, but they are circles. So the suturing has to be like the rays of the sun. Since it is a circle, there is no angle, so there is no angle of sorrow. The angle of sorrow arises only because from one end of the suture to the other, you make parallel bites. There are only four places where you should hold the needle at right angles, i.e., at the edges. The rest of the time, your needle should be at a slight angle. Your wrist movement remains the same, though the direction of the needle changes.

A problem that all of us face at some point is how to take bites at a depth. The place is deep. Take your hand in there that way and then your bite. You will find it easy. Do not hold it like this. Hold it this way. There is no harm. Always use a long needle holder. Hold it, go down to the depth that you need to with your thread and take the bite as precisely as you want. Learn to hold it the way you hold a pen and when you reach the site then rotate. These are skills for people who operate deep inside the pelvis or cystic duct. You sometimes need to take a bite where you cannot get your hand in. Learn to take a bite with your left hand. Another important thing you need to practice is to support the needle when you take it out and then take the clip the way you are going to use it for your next bite. Otherwise, you will waste a lot of time when you are going around an anastomosis, for example. This is why some surgeons take less time than others. So, get into the habit of holding your needle the way you are going to use it for the next bite. If you are going to change direction then hold it in reverse, so that you are ready for the next bite. These may seem like small things, but they all add up. If you keep fiddling around, it is going to break. So, whenever you are doing that deliberately try to hold it for your next bite. The angle, the direction, because if your previous bite is right, the next one is bound to be right. The tissues fall together.

Right Forceps

Next we come to holding tissue with forceps. that for dissecting what we tend to use put forceps for suturing skins or holding the skin when you are making subcutaneous tissue, You must use the appropriate forceps to prevent the needle from turning and it keeps getting bent because it is not meant to hold this. So, use the appropriate instruments. When you are using fine needles then please use fine instruments and specially designed forceps suited to the size of the needle that you are using. Otherwise, the needle will get flattened and lose its shape. And do not hold the suture in the middle, just at the tips.

Uneven Edges

When you are trying to bring together edges that are uneven in size, you will keep cheating or taking more of one and less of the other. If you want to make it smooth, then you have to accommodate this much in that much. The jaws of a needle holder or artery forceps should appose by the second ratchet. After that, it is just a question of applying pressure. If the jaws do not come together by the second ratchet, then the needle holder is not good. You should be able to hold your hair with artery forceps by the second ratchet. The last one is just to add pressure. A needle holder is ideally supported by the right ring finger. The middle finger has nothing to do with it. Use these two fingers. Essentially this is your movement. You have to always support it. So, the bite is important, but the throw is more important. Every throw has got to hold. And you duplicate with your left had what you do with your right.

Appropriate Needle

If you use a blunt or a round-body needle to go through the thickest skin, say in the sole of the foot or the back of the head, it is not going to work. Or you take on the face great big beautiful taper cut and reverse cutting making the surface horrible! Using the appropriate-sized needle and instruments is very important. If you have got the right needle you do not need to apply undo pressure. I do an entire transplant with no tooth forceps, no tooth instrument of any kind. If you ask the assistant to hold the needle and with an artery forceps, the needle lost somewhere, having bleeding, etc.

Distance of Bite

What should be the distance of the bite from the edge of the skin and what should be the distance between bites? In general, the thickness of the bite should be proportionate to the thickness of the structure you are going through. Take for example the skin, you cannot have bites of 1 mm unless you are a plastic surgeon and you know what you are trying to achieve. But in general, the skin itself is about two-thirds of a centimeter thick. If you are going to take breath bites the whole thing will come out. Roughly, the thickness of the skin should be the distance from the edge, and also the distance between two bites. In the case of an artery or vein, the bites should be 1 mm apart and 1 mm from the edge. But if you do the same in the bowel, you will devascularize it; 1 mm is too close. In vascular anastomosis, the mucosa must evert, but in the bowel, the mucosa must be inward. If you evert a bowel anastomosis, you will get a leak. So, each anastomosis has its own requirement. If you have to force the needle through, you are using the wrong material. The needle should always glide through.

Lastly, these days we do not use needles without threads. However, you should all learn how to thread a needle because there may be occasions when you require a needle without a thread. You must learn how to thread it with this on the needle holder.

Stumps

Harsha Jauhari

■ INTRODUCTION

A vast majority of surgical disasters occur due to errors related to the stump. They are pulled off, the gap comes away, the ties loosen, and it gets blown off disasters occur around stumps. Your assistant does not tie it well or you do not tie it well, the coordination is not good. All in all, stumps are the tombstones under which lie the buried, many a surgical reputation.

What is the ideal length of a stump? It should be one and a half times the diameter beyond the tie for it to be safe. Anything less will slip out, anything long is unnecessary.

A stump may contain arteries, veins, ureters, nerves, and tissue—each needs a different approach. An artery, by its nature, has adventitia, a muscular layer and an intimal layer. It is round. A vein, on the other hand, is a flat, thin structure. You cannot tie the two in the same way. If you do, you are asking for trouble so, they all need a different approach. If you tie an artery too tight, you will slice through the intima and the muscular layer in an atherosclerotic patient, and all you will be left with is the adventitia and suddenly the whole thing will blow. Similarly, you should not tie a single suture on an artery because there will be a pressure of 140 mm Hg hammering away at the suture and it may give way, unless you are the kind of person who ties his knots perfectly. Remember that you are bunching up the circumference into a very small area, so ideally, you should double ligate, or even triple ligate, sometimes. The most distal one, against which the pressure builds up, will blow first. So, you tie the next one below it and then the third one because this is the one that is going to keep everything safe. Once the artery has been empty then you tie it. A vein, on the other hand, is a flat ribbon. You are trying to tie it into a circle. So, you have to give yourself enough length of vein for allowing me to bunch out. Tying it once is enough, except in the case of major veins. Ureters and nerves are solid, so you can tie them without much trouble. Do not tie too tightly, or there will be leaks. The tie has to be firm, but not so strong as to devascularize the whole thing.

If you have to tie up a major artery (e.g., an iliac artery), you do a transfixion ligation. It may be difficult to clamp something at right angles to the structure, especially in the case of a bulky stump. There will always be a drift below the clamp. If you have to transfix, do it on the shorter side, not on the longer side. Secure the shorter side to prevent slipping. If you transfix the longer side, it is going to slip. This is the cause of all bleedings. Never pull the knot upwards at an angle because the force then acts outward and the knot slips. This should be clear if you recall the parallelogram of forces. The only way to tighten the knot is in the straight line. Place your fingers close to the knot and tighten it on the knuckles **(Fig. 1)**. Do not try to tighten

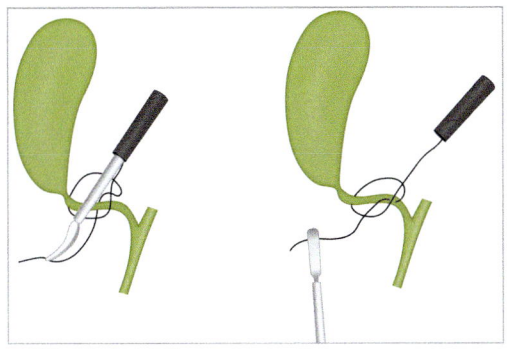

Fig. 1: Knotting the cystic duct.

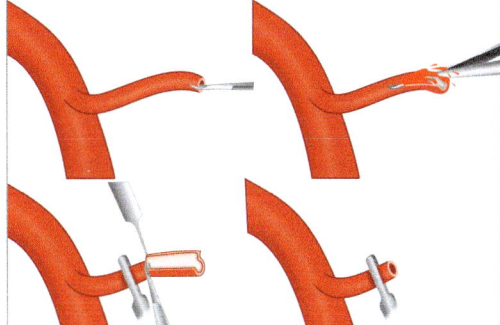

Fig. 2: Preparation of an arterial stump.

from a distance. If the knot is giving in, you must make it more snug, and let it progress to the adequate tightness. Each fiber has its own compressibility and needs to settle down with each other. There is no hurry. Ensure that both edges are visible within the suture loop. Take the loop of the knot as far down as you can. Spending a few extra seconds on this particular step is going to save you a lot of grief. There is an old saying that you must point the tip of the hemostat towards the surgeon's nose. Apply the hemostat correctly tip pointing upwards, not necessarily in the direction of your surgeon or your assistant, to make sure that he gets to see the tip. Tilt it in one direction and then another, if need be. There is another tip that I would like to share. Surgeons tend to look away when they have finally got everything right, and it is just a matter of tightening. They let their fingers guide them. Rely on your fingers when everything is in place and it is virtually the last millimeter or two. Your fingers will tell you whether you have made it too tight or too loose or just right. And especially with major vessels. Now, first make your proper knot, then go for the second one. Because you do not have a second chance. First bite is always the best. Any major artery, any major vein, never create suction on the knot. Tying an artery has to be close to the origin as possible.

Preparation of the arterial stump is a very intricate procedure before anastomosis in vascular surgery **(Fig. 2)**. This is for all major vascular surgeries and particularly for Liver and Renal transplant surgeries **(Fig. 3)**.

By and large, it is not a good idea to have broad stumps. If it is necessary then place the clamp as low as possible, dissect and break the tissue bulk into smaller structures. Short stumps are problematic, but you have to deal with them sometimes, for example, close to the aorta. Do not be in a hurry. If you have to make a single tie around a short and broad stump, should you tighten at the short end or the broad side? The weakest part of a knot is where you have tied it because it is not smooth. The smoothest part is the opposite side. So, secure the short side always or it will slip on that side. If you have to tighten the knot, do so at the longer side, not the shorter side.

Sometimes when you are tying a knot at a depth, the tissue may retract. Get your sutures, get your suctions. Take a bite through any edge or corner of the stump that you can find. But do not tie the knot just yet. If you can get the other edge with a slight traction, take another bite. Dig in your needle and pull it out. It is alright even if you get half a bite. Get as many of them as possible. Do not tie the knots. Hold all of them in your hand and with your artery, clamp it and

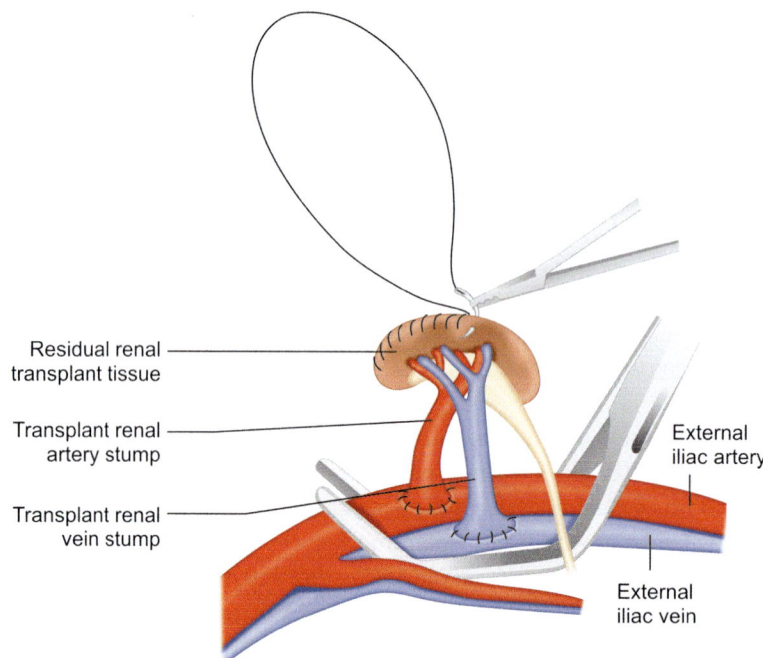

Fig. 3: The renal stumps in transplant surgery.

God willing, it will hold. You may gain 2 or 3 mm; that is all you require. It will save the patient. Only you can do this because only you have the coordination required. You know when you are going to pull and you know when you are going to let go. Even if you have got half the stump, you can repeat the maneuver. Remember never to tie the knot right away after the first bite.

Deep, unapproachable and awkward stumps require better light, better approach and better technique. Do not take chances. Never compromise the stumps. That is the basic motto. A very tight stump is a "leakpost." If you feel that the knot is too tight, you may have to be back at the operating table within the next few hours or on the next day for damage control.

When you tie a stump that is clamped across by artery forceps, you tie the knot at the edge. So when you start tightening it, it will slip off. The moment the forceps comes off, it will just slip off. To prevent this, make sure that the knot lies at the side of the stump, not at the apex or the base, so that the distance on both sides is equal. This reduces the chances of the knot slipping off. Even when you transfix, for example, in the case of the uterine stump, you got the uterine vessels, you got the broad ligament, and things coming off, you got a fairly broad base, and you got it literally on the curved artery forceps on the uterus. If you pull the thread up and tie a knot, as you keep tightening, it will keep slipping and suddenly the knot will slip completely off the stump. Another thing you must remember when you are doing a transfixation is that you must do it on the short side. This way you have the whole length and width to play with.

If the stump has a broad base and includes important structures, make the transfixation on the important structure, rather than on the whole bunch of tissues. Trying to transfix an artery in the stump may result in a big hematoma, so transfixing an artery is not a good idea. When you have got it under control, with mosquito forceps, dissect and take the vessel separately from the rest of the tissues. Taking a blind bite may work 9 times out of 10, but one out of 10 times you may hit the artery and have a hematoma with a lot of tissue around it. The way to tackle a stump is to make it as bare as possible and as safe as possible and to not poke needles into it if you can avoid it. Very few pedicles will be big enough to require to be transfixed. You may need to do it only in an emergency. For example, in an emergency nephrectomy, the entire pedicle may need to be clamped and ligated because of massive bleeding, but even in that situation, it is advisable to clamp first and then look below to see if you can tie the knot separately on the artery.

Tying a knot is more than just tying a knot. It is something you do to have a comfortable night's sleep. You do not want to leave the stump in such a condition that it might blow. Surgery is executed on the table, but it is practiced at home, and imagined in your mind. Learn about needles, needle holders, artery forceps and knots, try and understand the theories behind these, and most importantly, observe and learn. A surgeon who does not change direction gets his knot wrong. Simply put, the entire surgical field depends on the knot, a proper reef knot.

■ CONCLUSION

Knots on a stump should be perfectly tied to prevent unnecessary complications in this critical part of surgery and prevent a potentially devastating dehiscence or stump blowout.

CHAPTER 18

Sutures and Suturing Techniques

Vasundhara Oberoi

■ INTRODUCTION

Tissues are sutured in situations in which they will not heal and regain strength, unless they are artificially approximated. The type of suture depends on the type of tissue, grade of contamination, cosmesis and most importantly, the surgeon's choice and experience.

"Size" denotes the diameter of the suture material. The size of the suture is stated numerically, as the number of zeroes in the suture size increases, the diameter of the strand decreases and the tensile strength also does. There are United States Pharmacopeia (USP) regulations, sutures thicker than the first size zero were calibrated onto whole numbers such as 1, 2, and so on.

■ TYPES OF SUTURE MATERIALS

- Absorbable
- Nonabsorbable
- Monofilament
- Polyfilament.
  Ideal suture material should have the following attributes:
- Adequate suture length.
- It should cause minimal tissue reaction.
- It should be easy to handle.
- The knotting quality should be good.
- It should be nonallergenic and non-carcinogenic.
- It should be easily available and cheap.
  Before using a suture, you should be aware of its characteristics and more importantly, of the information on the packaging.

Keep the following in mind:
- Take note of the number. The first suture was "0". As the number of zeroes increases, the suture becomes finer.
- Check for the length of the suture in centimeter.
- Silk is best kept dry.
- Nylon should be drawn to remove memory.

TYPES OF SUTURING TECHNIQUES

- Ligatures are sutures that are tied around vessels. They can be used for a free tie or a stick tie, in the case of deep bleeding.
- Primary suture lines are of the following types:
  - *Continuous sutures*: With this suture, you should guard against overtightening and exercise caution in cases of infection.
  - *Interrupted sutures*: These can be simple or mattress sutures and are more secure.
  - *Purse string sutures*: These are used to tighten lumens such as the appendix stump.
  - *Subcuticular sutures*: These are dermal in nature.
- *Secondary suture line*: This reinforces primary closure, in secondary or delayed closure.
- *Retention sutures:* These are placed 2″ from the margin.
- *Through and through sutures*: These go through all layers including the peritoneum. They should be nonabsorbable in nature.

KNOTS

The tensile strength is measured by the force, in pounds, which the suture strand can withstand before it breaks when knotted.

- The characteristics of sutures that are relevant to knots are as follows:
  - "Hand" refers to the feel of the suture in the surgeon's hand.
  - Extensibility is the elasticity it offers when tying a knot.
  - Memory is the ability of the suture to fold over itself.
  - This must be released prior to tying a knot.
- Knots should be firm and should not slip. They should be small. Make sure you place them away from critical structures and avoid manhandling the sutures. Do not overtighten them and strangulate the tissue. The number of knots depends on the type of suture.
- The commonly used knots are the square knot; the friction knot, which is the most universal and is tied with monofilament sutures prone to slipping; and the deep tie, a square knot used at a deeper plane.

Absorbable suture: These are used when the tissue gets repaired and strength is regained faster than the loss of the suture's tensile strength. They are of the following two types:

- *Natural absorbable*: Catgut and chromic catgut sutures fall in this category. They have the following characteristics:
  - They are derived from the submucosa of sheep gut.
  - They are absorbed by the enzymatic process.
  - There is 50% loss of tensile strength in 3 days and 100% in days. Chromic lasts 30% longer than catgut.
  - These sutures are used for subcutaneous approximation in the oral region and lips; and in the bowel, muscles and peritoneum.
- *Synthetic absorbable*: These may be monofilament sutures.

TABLE 1: Absorbable sutures.

Polymer	Name	Loss of tensile strength	Advantage/disadvantage
Catgut	Plain/chromic	7–10 days	Cheap; rapid loss of tensile strength
Polyglactin	Vicryl	6–14 days	Expensive

TABLE 2: Delayed absorption.

Polymer	Name	Loss of tensile strength	Advantage/disadvantage
Polyglecaprone	Monocryl	120 days	Difficult to knot
Polydioxanone	PDS II	60 days	Strong and easy to handle

TABLE 3: Nonabsorbable sutures.

Polymer	Brand names	Feature
Silk	Mersilene	Braided; risk of infection
Stainless steel	Ethisteel	Strong; difficult to knot and handle
Polyamide	Ethilon	Less reactive; difficult to knot
Polyester	Ethibond	Slippery and difficult to knot
Polypropylene	Prolene	Easy to pass through tissue; difficult to knot; irritant to tissue

■ SUTURES AND SUTURING

Sutures may be absorbable or non absorbable. Absorbable sutures may bethose that have an early and those with delayed absorption **(Tables 1 to 3)**. [Polydioxanone (PDS); Monocryl] or polyfilament sutures (Vicryl). They have the following characteristics:
- Natural or colored
- Twice the strength of catgut
- Absorbed by hydrolysis
- Ethylene oxide sterilization
- Longer tensile strength.

The sutureless techniques are as follows:
- *Glue*: Cyanoacrylate (Dermabond) is a topical skin adhesive. It is a sterile skin adhesive that holds skin margins together. The film stays in place for 5–10 days, then falls of the skin.
- *Adhesive tapes (Ethistrip)*: These are used for approximating the edges of lacerations, skin closure, repair, and support in selected operative procedures. They are associated with minimal tissue reactivity and the lowest rate of infection. Their advantages include the fact that they can be applied rapidly, are inexpensive, and do not cause much discomfort to the patient. There is no risk of needle stick injuries or of suture hatch marks, so they can be allowed to remain for a longer time.

- *Surgical staples*: Staple closure is used mainly for large wounds that are not on the face. They are useful for linear laceration of the torso, scalp, and extremities. Staples are easy to use, can be applied rapidly, are cost-effective and cause minimal damage to the host's defense.
- *Zipline*: This is a rapid noninvasive skin closure device that eliminates staples, glue, and sutures. It offers a uniform closure pressure, creates an isolation zone around incision protecting it from patient-induced distraction forces, and cosmesis and closure speed are other advantages.

The sizes of sutures are determined by regulations laid down by the USP and indicated by the number of zeros. Originally, the thinnest suture available was designated number one (#1). As manufacturing techniques improved and sutures became thinner, zeros were added to denote the diameters of sutures. Thus, the greater the number of zeros, the thinner is the suture. For example, the #1 catgut suture has a diameter of 0.5–0.59 mm, the #0 collagen suture has a diameter of 0.4 mm, and the #10-0 (10 zeros) Ethilon suture, used by plastic surgeons and ophthalmic surgeons, has a diameter of just 0.2 mm. Remember that the diameter of a suture is not uniform throughout its length; it may vary within a range. Also, sutures of the same number but made of different materials may have different ranges of diameter; for example, a #1 nonabsorbable suture is thinner than a catgut suture of the same number, and has a diameter of 0.4–0.49 mm.

◼ CHOOSING THE TYPE OF SUTURE

How do you decide on the type of suture that you should use? Your decision should depend on the type of tissue, on how fast you expect it to heal and regain its strength and on the presence of foreign bodies and potential contamination. Similarly in luminal structures like urinary tract and biliary tract, if contaminants or foreign materials are present, do not use nonabsorbable sutures, which are permanent. If contaminants or foreign materials are present, do not use nonabsorbable sutures, which are permanent. If cosmesis is important, use fine sutures and remove them early. Sutureless tissue approximation has become common these days. Skin glues are used extensively. However, for this technique to be successful, the surface of the wound must be dry. Also, it only approximates the epidermis, you cannot use it deep inside the dermis. You have to suture the subdermal layer that will support the glue. Tapes may substitute skin suturing and help approximate the edges, but they cannot support the wound. Absorbable staples made of Vicryl can be used instead of sutures, but they are not commonly used because they are expensive.

◼ SUTURING TECHNIQUES

The first thing you must learn about suturing is where to enter the wound. The distance of the point of entry of the needle from the wound edge should be equal to the thickness of the skin (epidermis + dermis). The distance between two sutures should be equal to the distance between the wound edge and the point of entry of the needle. Hence, you should make a square and also the needle should enter the skin at 90°, and not at an acute angle. You must use more of the subcutaneous bulk, rather than the superficial tissue, while suturing to prevent "inversion" of the wound. Common suturing techniques include:

- The simple interrupted suture follows the same pattern
- Continuous or "over and over" running stitch are of two kinds. The commonly used one is "the simple continuous running stitch" that has a slanted appearance. It is the first method of skin closure. You must throw the needle at 90° to the movement to get an oblique line while suturing.
- The interrupted vertical mattress suture helps in relieving tension in the suture line and results in better approximation
- The horizontal mattress stitch is another technique which is used to reduce tension along the suture line. The disadvantage of this technique is that it being a complete square, between the sutures, the entire tissue can undergo ischemic necrosis.
- The purse-string suture is commonly used for anchoring drains.
- In subcuticular stitching, the most important layer which gives strength to the wound is the dermis, not the epidermis. Hence, you must approximate the dermis. It is not the fat or subcutaneous tissue which will help in wound repair healing. The advantage of this technique is that it minimizes scarring.

■ SOME IMPORTANT POINTS

- Apply surgical tapes across the wound at interrupted points and remove them from both sides. Do not pull across the wound because it may get disrupted.
- It is of paramount importance to delineate the area where you want to make the incision and to decide how to suture.
- The gentle handling of tissues cannot be overemphasized. Using a skin hook is important.
- Make the surface clear for the surgeon to operate, actually showing the underlying structures separately from the skin.
- If you use a subcuticular or subdermal stich to approximate the wound edges, you may not even require to apply a skin stitch and to achieve adequate hemostasis.

■ CONCLUSION

Tissue handling should be gentle and cannot be overemphasized.

■ SUGGESTED READING

1. Regula CG, Yag-Howard C. Suture Products and Techniques: What to Use, Where, and Why. Dermatol Surg. 2015;41(Suppl 10): S187-200.
2. Singer AJ, Hollander JE, Quinn JV. Evaluation and management of traumatic lacerations. N Engl J Med. 1997;337:1142-8.
3. Singer AJ. Lacerations and Acute Wounds: An Evidence-based Guide, 1st edition. Philadelphia: FA Davis Company; 2003.

Drains and Tubes

Ashish Dey

■ INTRODUCTION

Drains are channels designed to let out blood, pus or other body fluids from surgical wounds or body cavities to prevent them from becoming a focus of infection. The use of drains has been contentious and it is important that drainage should be practiced with prudence. Drains can be problematic if they are not selected properly, or if left *in situ* for too long. Of course, drains are not a substitute for good hemostasis and precise and meticulous surgical technique. Useful as they may be, they can cause more problems than they prevent. Drains can be active or passive and open or closed.

■ TYPES OF DRAINS

Passive Drains

These act by the mechanism of capillary action, gravity, or pressure differentials. The corrugated rubber drain, Penrose drain, and sump drain are some examples. Corrugated drains are flat, but have internal "ribs" to prevent them from collapsing or kinking.

Active Drains

These are tube drains that are aided by active suction, which could be continuous or intermittent. A few examples are the Jackson–Pratt drain **(Fig. 1)**, Biovac drain and Romovac drain. With these drains, it is possible to make a reliable measurement of the effluent. There is a decreased risk of wound infection and no skin excoriation.

It is to be noted that regular activation of the reservoir of the drain is often required. High-pressure drains can injure body tissues. These drains can also get clogged with tissue.

Open Drains

These drains empty directly to the exterior, into the overlying wound dressings or stoma bag. Corrugated rubber drains, Penrose drains, gauze wick drains and glove finger drains are a few examples. An open drain is used mostly for superficial wounds and cavities. It is simple and easy to apply. However, it is often difficult to measure the effluent.

Closed Drains

These are hollow tubes made of different materials. They are brought out through a body orifice or stab wound and are connected to a closed drainage system comprising a sterile drainage bag. The underwater seal drainage system is an example.

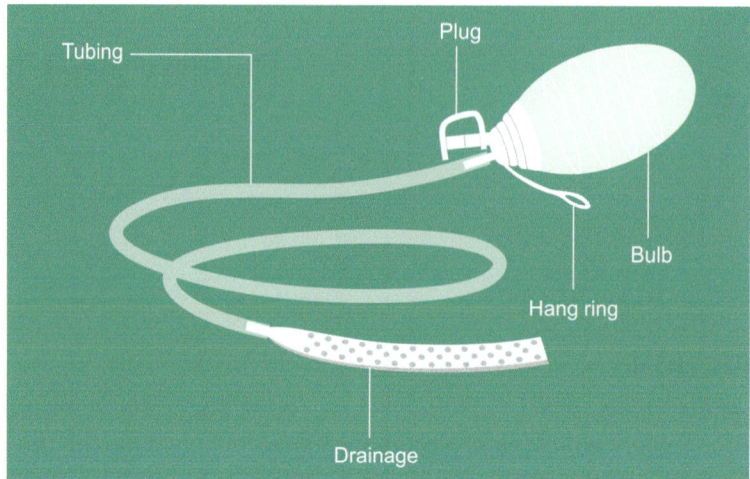

Fig. 1: Jackson–Pratt drain.

Some drains are made of materials that irritate the tissue and thus, can excite fibrous tissue response, leading to fibrosis and track formation. Some such materials are latex, plastic and rubber. Red rubber drains induce an intense tissue reaction that leads to the formation of a tract. In some situations, this may be helpful (e.g., biliary T-tube). Inert drains do not irritate the tissue and thus, ideally do not provoke tissue fibrosis. Some examples of such drains are polyvinyl chloride (PVC) and silicone drains.

■ COMPLICATIONS

Drains can cause complications such as anastomotic breakdown and hernias at the site of the drain. In the case of firm drains, erosion into hollow organs may occur.

■ REMOVAL

Generally, drains should be removed once the drainage has stopped or becomes <25 mL/day. You can "shorten" the drain by withdrawing it by approximately 2 cm/day, allowing the site to heal gradually. Drains that protect postoperative sites from leakage form a tract and are usually kept in place for 1 week.

■ SPECIAL DRAINS AND SPECIAL SITUATIONS

- Kehr's "T" tube is used for short-term postoperative drainage of the common bile duct.
- The chest tube, also known as an underwater sealed drain, is connected to a closed drainage system. It is used to drain the hemothorax, pneumothorax, chylothorax, pleural effusion and empyema.
- The pigtail drain has several uses. One of these is to allow urine to drain directly from a kidney if the ureter is diseased or blocked.
- The Redivac drain (a closed drain) is a fine tube with many holes at the end. It is attached to an evacuated glass bottle that provides suction. It is used to drain blood from beneath the skin, e.g., after a mastectomy or thyroidectomy or from deep spaces, such as around a vascular anastomosis.

■ IDEAL DRAIN

A drain should be firm enough to remain in its intended position. A very soft drain may twist or kink and get blocked. It should be smooth so that the bowel and other important structures do not adhere to it. A drain should be easy to remove later. It should be sufficiently narrow or wide and the lumen should be wide enough to prevent easy blockage. An ideal drain does not exist in practice, but an effort should be made to choose the most appropriate one in each situation.

■ PURPOSES OF DRAINS

- *Therapeutic*: A drain permits the exit of liquid and could be used to treat hydrocephalus and abscess cavities.
- *Palliative*: Drains can be used as a palliative measure to bypass a luminal obstruction.
- *Diagnostic*: An example of the diagnostic uses of drains is in postcholecystectomy T-tube cholangiograms when stones are retained in the common bile duct.
- *Monitoring*: An example is the use of a nasogastric tube to monitor progress in a patient with upper gastrointestinal bleeding.

Postoperative Care of a Surgical Drain

It is important to insert an external drain through a stab wound and not the main wound. Skin care is essential around the drain site to prevent infection and skin irritation. Changes in the character or volume of the fluid must be monitored and any complication resulting in the leakage of fluid must be identified as soon as possible. The drain container or reservoir should be emptied at least once a day and regular activation of the reservoir of active drains must be ensured.

When to Discontinue a Surgical Drain

Generally, a drain should be removed once the drainage has stopped, or the output has become <25–50 mL/day or when it has stopped serving the desired purpose. But, of course, the removal of the drain should depend on its intended purpose, the organ involved and the surgery performed. Apart from the volume of the drainage fluid, its color, character and viscosity must be considered before removing the drain.

■ CONTROVERSIES

The use of drains in surgical practice has been contentious.

The arguments in support of their use include the fact that they may allow for the early detection of anastomotic leaks or hemorrhage. Those who argue against their use assert that the presence of drains in the body increases the risk of infection, delays tissue healing, causes tissue damage due to mechanical pressure or suction, and may actually induce an anastomotic leak. The old dictum, "when in doubt, drain," no longer holds good. Drains are not innocuous when left *in situ* and may result in unnecessary complications when left for too long. Now, the dictum for abdominal surgeries is, "when in doubt, do not drain." You must be very alert and diligent about the follow-up. No single policy need to be followed dogmatically. You should consider each situation on its own merit and take care to select the appropriate drain. The routine use of drains may be abandoned in uncomplicated surgeries such as thyroid surgery. Drains should not provide a false sense of security and are not a substitute for adequate hemostasis and good surgical technique.

Dressings

Vasundhara Oberoi

■ INTRODUCTION

From leaves to medicinal herbs to hydrocolloids, the art of wound management has evolved through a long journey of evaluating knowledge and applying the best practices. Interestingly, almost everything that has ever been used as a dressing has stayed on, and new technologies have simply been added.

■ HEALING OF A WOUND

The first stage in the healing of a wound is the inflammatory phase, in which there is an abundance of leukocytes, platelets, and macrophages. Once hemostasis is achieved, the proliferative phase starts, with the multiplication of fibroblasts and platelets and release of growth factors. Lastly, the wound remodels in accordance with the requirement of the parent tissue and environmental factors. Platelets and fibroblasts combine to bring lots of growth factors such as platelet-derived growth factors (PDGFs) and platelet-derived angiogenesis factor (PDAF). They along with epidermal growth factor (EGF) and transforming growth factor (TGF) along with essential micronutrients and vitamins C, D, and E help to form healthy granulation tissue. These can now be sourced through tissue engineering and used in wounds arrested at different stage of healing.

Table 1 differentiates between a contaminated wound and an infected wound.

To prevent the infection of a wound, you should reduce cross contact, monitor personal hygiene, use a clean dressing, prevent soiling by urine and ensure proper disposal of biowaste. In the event that a wound gets infected, the principles of management you should keep in mind are: proper debridement, preventing the formation of dead space and preemptive use of

TABLE 1: Differences between a contaminated and an infected wound.	
Contaminated wound	*Infected wound*
Almost all wounds	Only some wounds
It has a very low bacterial load	It has a very high bacterial load
It will heal	It will not heal
There is an abundance of exudate, which is rich in WBCs, lymphocytes, and growth factors.	There are systemic and local indicators such as fever and erythema, and deep tissue and blood culture may be positive.

drains when applicable. You should also use systemic and topical antibiotics judiciously and avoid using hydrogen peroxide and povidone iodine as these are anticellular.

■ DRESSING MATERIAL AND TECHNIQUE

The dressing material and technique you use are of paramount importance in ensuring a successful outcome.

Ideal dressing: The ideal dressing should be moist, cosmetic, biocomposite, leakproof, cheap, and odorless. It should facilitate gaseous exchange.

Bioelectric field: The generation of a bioelectric field is useful in the healing of a wound. A bioelectric field attracts cells, changes cell permeability, improves phagocytosis, encourages the growth of fibroblasts, and vasculogenesis. Wounds should be kept moist, which is why hydrogel dressings are important.

Uncovered wounds: Fistulae, areas of skin sealants, stage 1 pressure ulcers, grade 1 burns and traumatic wounds such as abrasions should not be covered.

Biodressings: These have several advantages. They are elastic, transparent, and durable. They maintain hydration and are nonantigenic, hemostatic, and provide bacterial barriers.

Negative pressure wound therapy: This involves the use of negative suction in a deep-pocketed wound with the help of a sponge and tight sealing. It helps by removing deleterious enzymes and edema, increases transudation, and hence activating platelets and blood vessel formation. They are not to be used in malignancies, ischemia, and inadequate debridement.

In summary, you have to choose the dressing technique and material in a scientific and prudent manner to optimize results **(Table 2)**.

What exactly is a dressing? Should we do a dressing? What should we dress and what we should use for the dressing? We all know the facts. So, you must first decide how you should do the dressing. For this you must examine the wound to find out whether it is contaminated or infected. Potentially, all wounds are contaminated. Your aim should be to prevent it from getting infected. A wound that contains exudate usually heals by itself. If you suspect an infection, the most important thing is to look at the culture report for sensitivity of the microorganisms.

A superficial swab culture may just pick up the contaminants. It is, therefore, important to do a tissue culture. Use forceps to pick up the sample, seal it off, and then send it to the laboratory. If you suspect an infection, a dressing will not suffice; you will need to treat it. You

TABLE 2: Dressing materials and their characteristics.		
Name of material	*Commercial name*	*Characteristics*
Alginate	Kaltostat	Nonwoven; seaweed; retains moisture
Hydrocolloid	Duoderm restore	Occlusive and adherent; absorbs exudate; good for granulation; no odor
Transparent fibers	Tegaderm, Opsite	Semipermeable; moist barrier; less friction
Collagen	Medfill, Skin temp, Kollagen	Easy to procure; good for hemostasis; encourages repair
Tissue engineered fibroblasts	Apligraf, Dermagraft	From newborn foreskin; has dermis and epidermis with all growth factors

may have to use topical and/or systemic antibiotics. If you are dealing with an abscess, merely covering it will not ensure drainage of the contents. Use Betadine and hydrogen peroxide very selectively for dressing. Betadine inhibits healing, or rather, retards it. Though it definitely reduces the bacterial load, it also inhibits the growth of cells and formation of granulation tissue. It reduces the exudate, which carries all the enzymes and antibiotics for healing.

An ideal surgical dressing should:
- Be biocompatible
- Provide a moist environment
- Protect the wound
- Be able to absorb all the exudate
- Maintain optimum temperature and gaseous exchange
- Be inexpensive

■ EXUDATE

Exudates are normal secretions of any wound. They contain ribosomal enzymes, WBCs, lymphocytes, and growth factors, all of which promote healing. The moist environment of the exudate provides a medium for the passage of the current generated by this system. The moment a trauma occurs—it could be anything from a scratch to a rib bone fracture—a current is generated to help in healing the wound. The current interacts with the cells to initiate repair. It causes changes in the permeability of the cell membrane and agitates the cells toward healing.

A moist wound helps healing by lowering the infection rate. It reduces the wound closure time, so you will need fewer dressings. To keep the wound moist, you may use a simple 0.9% saline solution. Try to maintain an optimal bioelectric charge. The occlusive dressings and hydrogel dressings available these days are helpful in this respect. Do not use the common antiseptic "dusting powder" because it delays healing. It causes the formation of a scab, under which the infection festers.

■ PREVENTION OF INFECTION

Some important points to remember are the following:
- Avoid cross-contamination
- Follow the handwashing protocol
- Use clean dressing supplies and sterile instruments
- Wear fresh gloves
- Follow strict waste disposal norms
- Protect the wound from urinary or fecal contamination.

■ WHEN TO DRESS A WOUND

Dressings are required—(i) after surgery, in the sterile environment of the operation theater, to prevent contamination of the surgical wound and (ii) after debridement of a wound that needs to be covered.

The following types of wounds do not need to be covered:
- Cutaneous fistula not caused surgically
- Stage-I pressure ulcer

- First-degree burns
- Wounds caused by trauma that do not require surgical closure or debridement (e.g., abrasion, friction burns, venipuncture, and arterial puncture sites).

We tend to dress such wounds, more for mental satisfaction than anything else, like a "first-aid" approach. Skin sealants or barriers, topical antiseptic, and enzymatic debriding agents do not need a cover.

FREQUENCY OF DRESSING A WOUND

How often you should dress a wound depends on the type of dressing you use.
- If you use alginates, change the dressing every day
- In the case of foam dressing, changing on alternate days should suffice.
- A gauze piece gets soaked easily, so change it twice or thrice a day
- Hydrogel and special absorptive dressings need to be changed once a day.

Adhesive transparent dressing:
- If you use transparent films, change the dressing every second day
- In the case of Steri-Strips, it is up to the surgeon to decide on the frequency of changing the dressing

TYPES OF DRESSINGS

Dressings are of two types—(1) synthetic and (2) biological. The former are hydrocolloid dressings. They are available in the form of gels, powders, and foams. You have to combine them before application. They absorb exudates from the wound and prevent them from leaking out. They also prevent the wound from getting contaminated from the outside. They are good for granulating wounds and they reduce pain. You may have heard of Duoderm, Restore, and Comfeel. These dressings are available in different shapes to match the contour of different sites of the body. Transparent films are semipermeable membrane dressings that help retain moisture. Some examples are Tegaderm and Opsite. They prevent contamination and do not adsorb exudates.

Biological dressings are ideal dressings. These nonhydrogenic, nontoxic, and nearly transparent dressings are easily available. They are hydrated and do not need tapes around them. They act as bacterial barriers, can be removed easily and allow the transfer of water vapor. Alginates, made of soft nonwoven fibers derived from seaweeds, are common biological dressings. They keep the wound moist, though they require a secondary dressing.

Collagen dressings, made from animal sources such as bovine hide, may be used even to cover burn wounds. They are hemostatic and hasten healing by stimulating fibroblasts to lay down collagen. What takes about 2 weeks, may be healed up within 7 days. Collagen dressings are available as powders, gels, sheets, and granules.

GRAFTS AND TISSUE ENGINEERING

What is a skin substitute? Skin substitutes may be homografts (which are basically skin grafts), heterografts, or amniotic membrane. They are temporary dressings to provide a temporary skin cover.

Tissue engineering, which is now gaining ground, is more like growing skin. Samples are taken from the patient in the form of human fibroblast. They can be the foreskin of newborn infants after circumcision. They may also be taken from human epidermal and dermal layers, so it is more durable.

■ PLATELET-DERIVED GROWTH FACTOR

We have not started using this yet, but it is available in western countries, though it is very expensive. Platelets derived from the patient's blood sample are put into storage containers. All you have to do is pour the solution over the wound. It contains PDGF, platelet-derived antigens, and platelet-derived EGF, other than the β-growth factor and platelet factor 4. All these help the process of healing.

However, there is no known substance that increases the rate of healing significantly. All you can do is to reduce the factors that prevent healing—prevent infection, deal with vitamin C deficiency, and protein deficiency. The acid-digested bovine cartilage powder has been shown to increase the rate of healing to an extent. However, it is nothing but collagen. On the whole, there is not much you can do to make a wound heal faster.

■ SUGGESTED READING

1. Baranoski S, Ayello EA. Wound dressings: An evolving art and science. Adv Skin Wound Care. 2012;25:87-92; quiz 92-4.
2. Landriscina A, Rosen J, Friedman AJ. Systematic approach to wound dressings. J Drugs Dermatol. 2015;14:740-4.
3. Lawrence CJ. Dressings and wound infection. Am J Surg. 1994;167:S21-4.

21 Knots and Knotting Techniques

Ashish Dey

■ INTRODUCTION

Surgery is as much art as it is science and technique. Dexterity and speed in tying knots correctly constitute an art which only practice can make perfect. Of the many knots described, only a few are used in the modern surgery. It is of paramount importance that each knot placed for approximation of tissues or ligation of vessels be perfectly made. It must hold and with proper tension.

Modern day surgeons have a wide choice of natural and synthetic suture materials. Ethicon, Inc. has brought out this Knot Tying Manual that teaches knot tying and handling of sutures and includes simplified and standardized suturing techniques. This is of course for the right-handed surgeons, who constitute the majority.

There are some simple guidelines for sutures and suturing. Multifilament sutures are generally easier to handle and to tie than monofilament sutures, however, all the synthetic materials require a specific knotting technique. With multifilament sutures, the nature of the material and the braided or twisted construction provide a high coefficient of friction and the knots remain as they are laid down. In monofilament sutures, on the other hand, the coefficient of friction is relatively low, resulting in greater tendency for the knot to loosen after it has been tied. In addition, monofilament synthetic polymeric materials possess the property of memory.

Suture knots must be properly placed to be secure. Speed in tying knots may result in less than perfect placement of the strands. Considerable variation may also be found between knots tied by different surgeons and even between knots tied by the same individual on different occasions. Uniformity is extremely important for good outcomes.

■ GENERAL PRINCIPLES OF KNOT TYING

Certain general principles govern the tying of all knots and apply to all suture materials, which are as follows:

- The completed knot must be firm, so that once tied slipping is virtually impossible.
- The knot must be as small as possible to prevent an excessive amount of tissue reaction when absorbable sutures are used, or to minimize foreign body reaction when nonabsorbable sutures are used. Ends should be cut as short as possible.

- In tying any knot, friction between strands, due to the "sawing" movement, must be avoided as this can weaken the integrity and strength of the suture.
- Care should be taken to avoid damage to the suture material when handling. Avoid the crushing application of surgical instruments, such as needle-holders and forceps to the strand, only except when grasping the tip of the free end of the suture, during an instrument tie.
- Excessive tension applied by the surgeon will cause breaking of the suture and may cut through the tissue. Also sutures used for approximation should not be tied too tightly, because this may contribute to tissue strangulation and poor outcomes.
- After the first loop is tied, it is necessary to maintain traction on one end of the strand to avoid loosening of the throw of the knot.
- Final tension on final throw should be as nearly horizontal as possible using the knuckles and not vertical, as it may make the knot come off the free end of the stump or loosen the knot. If the two ends of the suture are pulled in opposite directions with uniform rate and tension, the knot may be tied more securely.
- Extra ties do not add to the strength of a properly tied knot. They only contribute to its bulk which must be avoided.

An important part of good suturing technique is correct method in knot tying. A seesaw motion, or the sawing of one strand down over another until the knot is formed, may materially weaken sutures. They may break when the second throw is made or, even worse, in the postoperative period when the suture is further weakened by increased tension or tissue edema.

■ SQUARE KNOT: TWO-HANDED

TABLE 1: Square knot: two-handed technique.

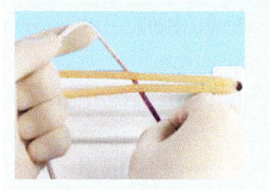 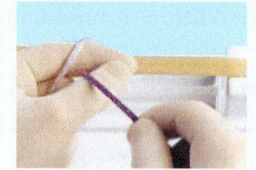 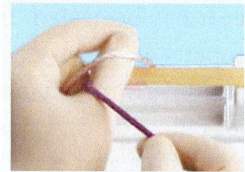 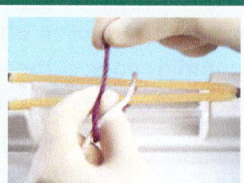

| 1. White strand is placed over extended index finger of the left hand acting as bridge and held in palm of the left hand. Purple strand is held in the right hand | 2. Purple strand is held in the right hand brought between the left thumb and index finger | 3. Left hand is turned inward by pronation and thumb swung under the white strand to form first loop | 4. Purple strand is crossed over white and held between the thumb and index finger of the left hand |

Contd...

Contd...

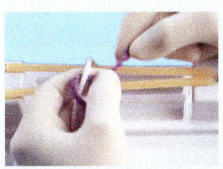

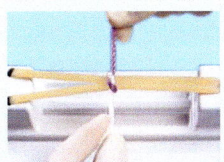

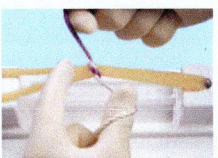

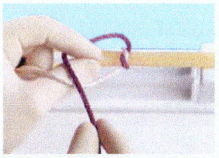

5. Right hand releases purple strand. Then left hand is supinated, with thumb and index finger still grasping purple strand, to bring purple strand through the white loop. Regrasp purple strand with the right hand

6. Purple strand is released by left hand and grasped by right. Horizontal tension is applied with the left hand toward and right hand away from the operator. This completes first half hitch

7. Left index finger is released from white strand and left hand again supinated to loop white strand over the left thumb

8. Purple strand is held in the right hand is angled slightly to the left. Purple strand is brought toward the operator with the right hand and placed between the left thumb and index finger. Purple strand crosses over the white strand

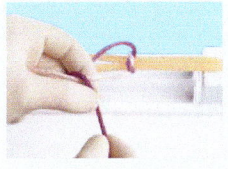

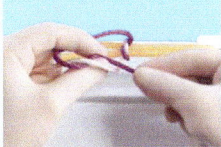

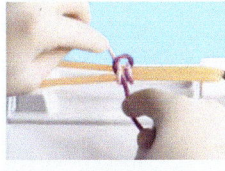

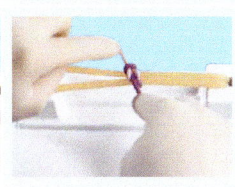

9. By further supinating left hand, white strand slides onto the left index finger to form a loop as purple strand is grasped between left index finger and thumb

10. Left hand is rotated inward by pronation with thumb carrying purple strand through loop of white strand. Purple strand is grasped between the right thumb and index finger

11. Horizontal tension is applied with left hand away from and right hand toward the operator. This completes the second half hitch

12. The final tension on the final throw should be as nearly horizontal as possible

■ SQUARE KNOT: ONE-HANDED

TABLE 2: Square knot: one-handed technique.

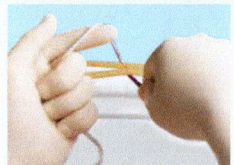 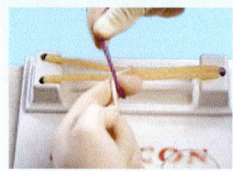 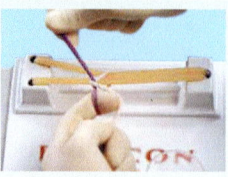 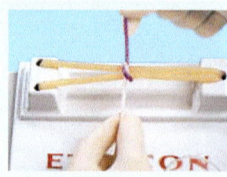

1. White strand is held between thumb and index finger of left hand with a loop over the extended index finger. Purple strand is held between the thumb and index finger of right hand	2. Purple strand is brought over white strand on left index finger by moving right hand away from the operator	3. With purple strand supported in right hand, the distal phalanx of left index finger passes under the white strand to place it over tip of left index finger. Then the white strand is pulled through loop in preparation for applying tension	4. The first half hitch is completed by advancing tension in the horizontal plane with the left hand drawn toward and right hand away from the operator

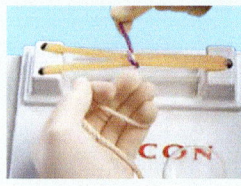 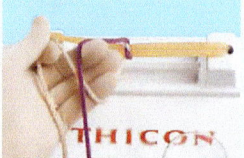 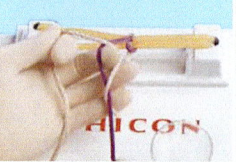 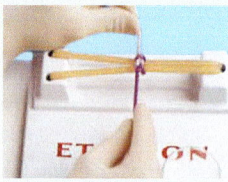

5. White strand is looped around three fingers of the left hand with distal end held between the thumb and index finger	6. Purple strand is held in right hand brought toward the operator to cross over the white strand. Continue hand motion by flexing distal phalanx of left middle finger to bring it beneath white strand	7. As the middle finger is extended and the left hand pronated, the white strand is brought beneath the purple strand	8. Horizontal tension is applied with the left hand away from and the right hand toward the operator. This completes the second half hitch of the square knot. Final tension should be as nearly horizontal as possible

■ SURGEON'S KNOT

TABLE 3: Surgeon's knot technique.

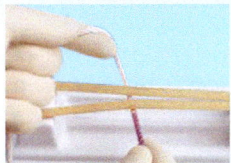

1. White strand is placed over the extended index finger of left hand and is held in palm of the left hand. Purple strand held between thumb and index finger of right hand

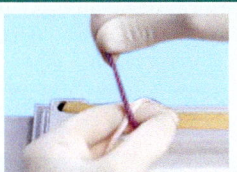

2. Purple strand is crossed over white strand by moving right hand away from the operator at an angle to the left. Thumb and index finger of left hand is pinched to form loop in the white strand over the index finger

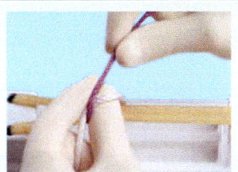

3. Left hand is turned inward by pronation, and loop of white strand is slipped onto left thumb. Purple strand grasped between thumb and index finger of left hand. Release right hand

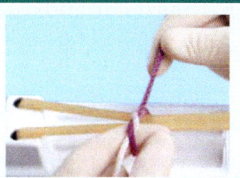

4. Left hand is rotated by supination extending left index finger to pass purple strand through loop. Regrasp purple strand with right hand

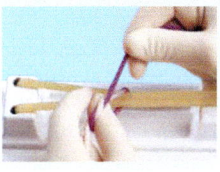

5. The loop is slid onto the thumb of the left hand by pronating the pinched thumb and index finger of left hand beneath the loop

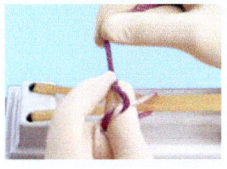

6. Purple strand is drawn left with right hand and again grasped between thumb and index finger of left hand

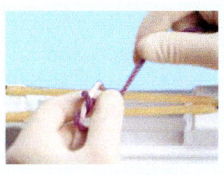

7. Left hand is rotated by supination extending left index finger to again pass purple strand through, forming a double loop

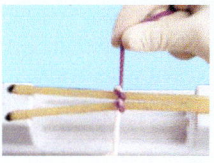

8. Horizontal tension is applied with left hand toward and right hand away from the operator. This double loop must be placed in precise position for the final knot

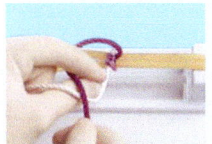

9. With thumb swung under white strand, purple strand is grasped between the thumb and index finger of left hand and held over white strand with right hand

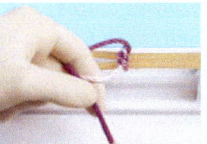

10. Purple strand released. Left hand supinates to regrasp purple strand with index finger beneath the loop of the white strand

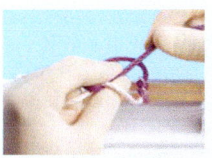

11. Purple strand rotated beneath the white strand by supinating pinched thumb and index finger of left hand to draw purple strand through the loop. Right hand regrasps purple strand to complete the second throw square

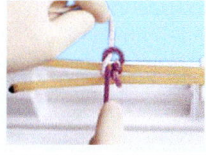

12. Hands continue to apply horizontal tension with left hand away from and right hand toward the operator. Final tension on final throw should be as nearly horizontal as possible

■ GRANNY KNOT

A granny knot is not recommended. However, it may be inadvertently tied by incorrectly crossing the strands of a square knot. It is shown only to warn against its use. It has the tendency to slip when subjected to an increasing pressure.

Deep Tie

TABLE 4: Deep tie technique.			
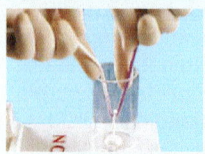	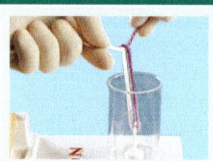	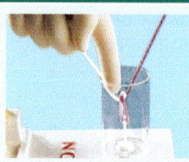	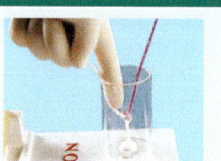
1. Strand looped around hook in plastic cup on Practice board with index finger of right hand which holds purple strand in palm of hand. White strand is held in left hand	2. Purple strand is held in right hand brought between the left thumb and index finger. Left hand is turned inward by pronation, and thumb swung under white strand to form the first loop	3. By placing index finger of left hand on white strand, advance the loop into the cavity	4. Horizontal tension is applied by pushing down on white strand with left index finger while maintaining counter tension with index finger of right hand on purple strand
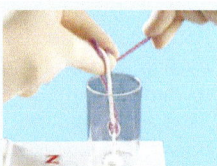	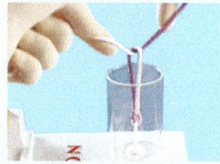	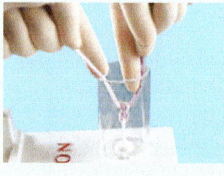	
5. Purple strand is looped over and under white strand with right hand	6. Purple strand is looped around white strand to form second loop. This throw is advanced into the depths of the cavity	7. Horizontal tension is applied by pushing down on purple strand with right index finger while maintaining counter tension on white strand with left index finger. Final tension should be as nearly horizontal as possible	

Tie with an Instrument

TABLE 5: Tie with an instrument.

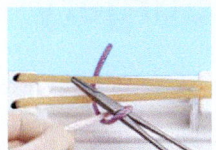

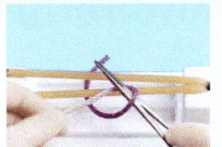

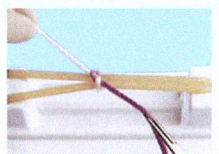

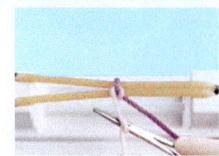

1. Short purple strand lies freely. Long white end of strand is held between the thumb and index finger of left hand. Loop is formed by placing needle holder on the side of strand away from the operator

2. Needle holder in right hand grasps short purple end of strand

3. First half hitch is completed by pulling needle holder toward operator with right hand and drawing white strand away from operator. Needle holder is released from the purple strand

4. First half hitch completed by pulling the needle holder toward operator with right hand and drawing white strand away from operator. Needle holder is released from the purple strand

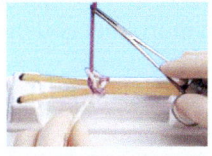

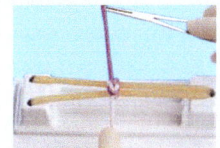

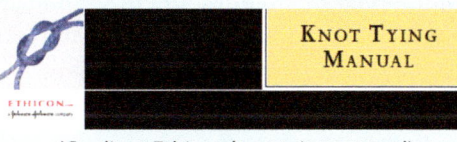

(Credits – Ethicon knot tying manual)

5. With end of the strand grasped by the needle holder, purple strand is drawn through loop in the white strand away from the operator

6. Square knot is completed by horizontal tension applied with left hand holding white strand toward operator and purple strand in needle holder away from operator. Final tension should be as nearly horizontal as possible

Source: Copied from - Knot tying manual, Ethicon Inc, USA', (Open access).

CHAPTER 22

Painting, Draping, and Positioning in Surgery

Rajesh Khullar

■ INTRODUCTION

Before the middle of the 19th century, surgical patients commonly developed postoperative infection, followed by purulent drainage from the incision, overwhelming sepsis and often, death. In late 1860, after Joseph Lister introduced the principle of antisepsis, postoperative sepsis decreased substantially.

The advances in infection control practices include improved ventilation of the operating room, sterilization methods, barrier surgical techniques and antimicrobial prophylaxis. Painting **(Fig. 1)**, draping, and positioning of patients are essential prerequisites of surgery. They significantly reduce infection at the surgical site, infection-associated morbidity and the burden of expenses borne by the patient.

Measures for the prevention of infection at the surgical site comprise a set of actions taken intentionally to reduce the risk of such infection.

■ PREOPERATIVE MEASURES

Antiseptic Showering

Preoperative antiseptic (chlorhexidine/povidone-iodine) showering does reduce microbial counts on the skin, but evidence suggests that it does not definitely reduce infection at the surgical site.

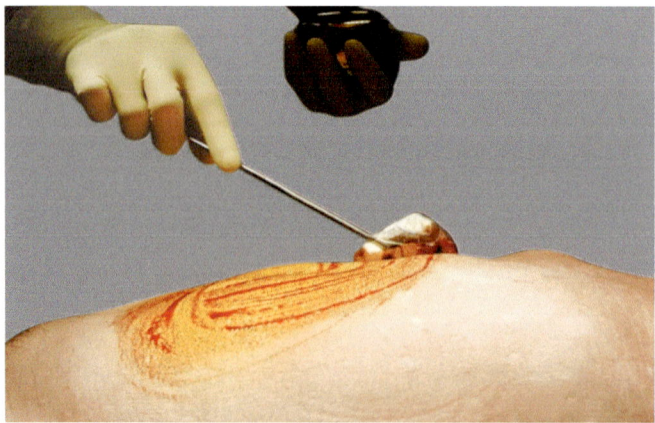

Fig. 1: Technique of painting the surgical site.

Hair Removal

Preoperative shaving of the surgical site the night before the surgery is associated with a significantly higher chance of infection than the use of depilatory agents or no hair removal. The increased risk of infection associated with shaving has been attributed to microscopic cuts in the skin that serve to multiply bacteria. Clipping the hair immediately before the surgery is associated with a lower chance of infection at the surgical site than shaving or clipping it the night before the surgery. Although the use of depilatories is associated with a lower risk of infection, they can produce hypersensitivity reactions. It has also been suggested that no method of hair removal is the best way of reducing infection.

Skin Preparation in Operating Room

Several antiseptic agents are available for preoperative skin preparation at the site of the incision. Povidone-iodine and products containing alcohol and chlorhexidine gluconate are the most commonly used agents. Alcohol is readily available, inexpensive, and the most effective and rapid-acting skin antiseptic. Aqueous (70–92%) alcohol solution has germicidal activity against bacteria, fungi, and viruses, but not spores. A potential disadvantage of the use of alcohol in the operating room is its flammability.

Both chlorhexidine gluconate and iodophors have broad spectra of antimicrobial activity. Chlorhexidine gluconate brings about a greater reduction in skin microflora than povidone-iodine. It also has greater residual activity after a single application. Chlorhexidine gluconate is not inactivated by blood or serum proteins. Iodophors may be inactivated by blood or serum proteins, but they exert a bacteriostatic effect as long as they are present on the skin. Before initiating skin preparation, the skin should be made free of gross contamination. The skin is prepared by applying an antiseptic in concentric circles, starting with the area of the proposed incision. The prepared area should be large enough to cover any extension of the incision or the creation of a new incision or drain site.

Surgical Draping

The procedure of covering a patient and surrounding the site of surgery with a sterile barrier to create and maintain a sterile field during a surgical procedure is called *draping*. The purpose of draping is to eliminate the passage of microorganisms from nonsterile areas to the sterile area. The procedure creates an area of asepsis, called a *sterile field*. Standard practice of draping includes the following:

- Only sterile drapes should be used within the sterile field.
- Drapes must be free of holes, punctures or tears.
- Drapes should be resistant to the penetration of fluid.
- They should be flame-resistant.
- Drapes made of a reusable woven fabric should have the same barrier characteristics as those made of a single-use nonwoven disposable fabric.

Surgical Positioning of Patients

The goal of surgical positioning is to allow for optimal visualization of, and access to, the surgical site **(Fig. 2)**. The patient should be positioned in such a way as to cause the minimum

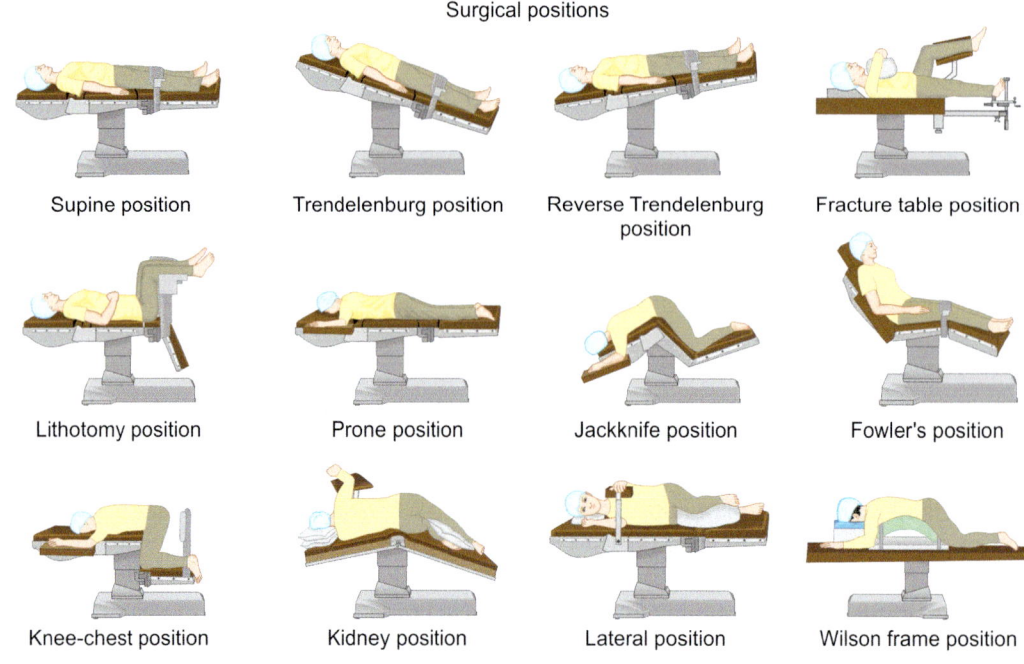

Fig. 2: Various positions in surgery.

physiological compromise and to protect the skin and joints. Once the patient has been administered anesthetic agents, he/she is no longer in the position to let the surgical team know if he/she is feeling pain or pressure. Therefore, the team becomes responsible for the patient. For this reason, the team must ensure that the patient has been positioned in a safe manner, and the functions of the integumentary, musculoskeletal, respiratory, and circulatory systems have been preserved.

Standard practice related to surgical positioning consists of the following.
- The surgical team should be familiar with the goals of achieving safe and effective positioning of the patient.
- During preoperative planning, surgeon, and other members of the surgical team should be informed about the patient's specific physiological factors that can affect the positioning procedure.
- On the basis of the preoperative assessment of the patient and the surgical procedure to be performed, the surgical technologist should determine the type of operating room table and equipment that is needed.
- The surgeon, in collaboration with the other members of the surgical team, should address the needs of special patient populations. They should take the precautions required to keep the patient from developing a pressure ulcer due to the surgical position.
- During preoperative planning for a surgical procedure, the surgeon and the other members of the surgical team should be informed if the patient is at particular risk of falling.

Finally, before performing the surgical scrub, the surgeon in the circulating assistant's role should assist in safely positioning the patient under the direct supervision of the chief surgeon and anesthesia care provider.

Vascular Anastomosis

Ajay Yadav

◼ INTRODUCTION

The principles of vascular repair with sutures were established in the first decade of the 20th century by Alexis Carrel.

Since then, suture materials have been technically refined to such an extent that it is now possible to surgically reconstruct most arteries, from the root of the aorta to microvascular anastomosis or repair of the smallest vessels. The use of atraumatic needles with fine sutures is the best for arterial anastomosis.

Joining two vessels or a vessel and graft is probably the most common major vascular procedure. The three different methods of doing this—(1) end-to-end, (2) end-to-side, and (3) side-to-side anastomoses—have very different applications **(Fig. 1)**.

Most of the commonly used techniques are described beneath. However, the experienced vascular surgeon often makes minor modifications, depending on the circumstances.

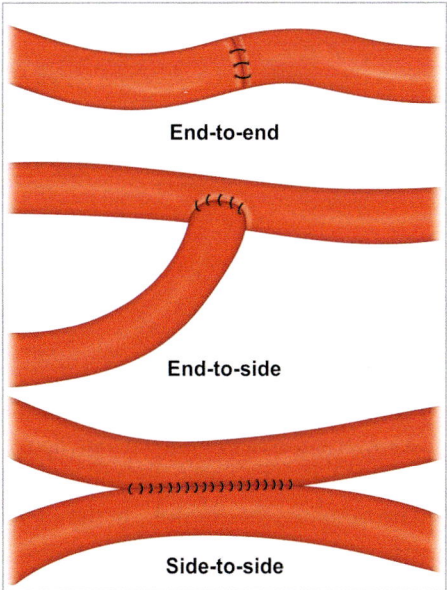

Fig. 1: Types of vascular anastomosis.

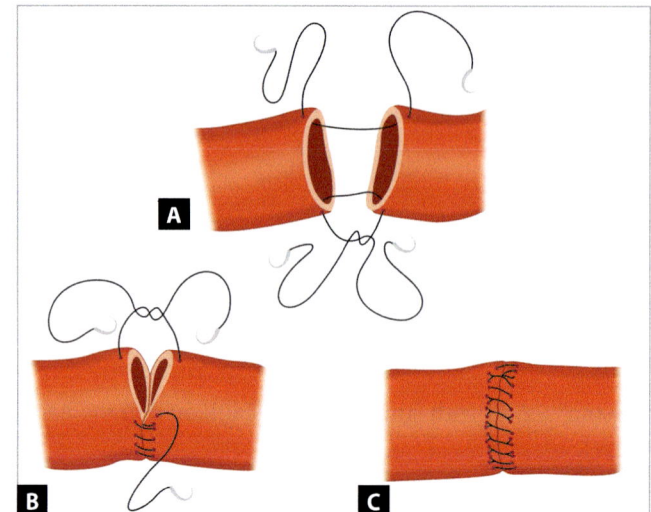

Figs. 2A to C: Simple perpendicular end-to-end anastomosis.

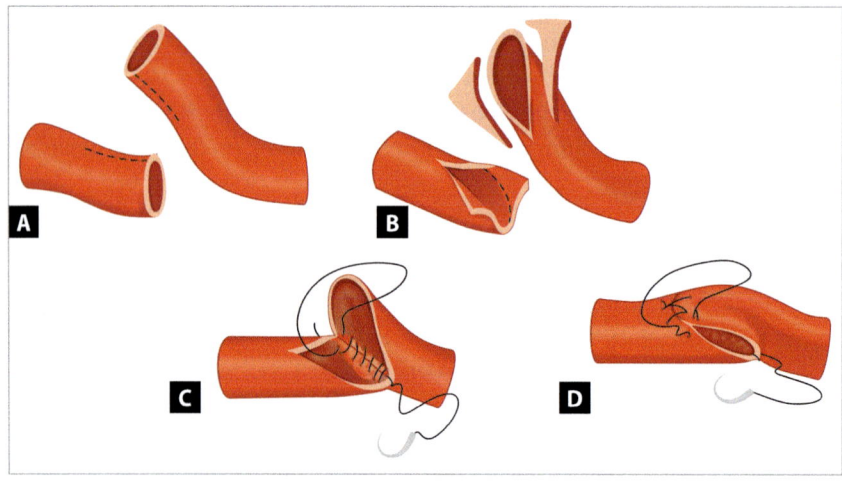

Figs. 3A to D: Technique of oblique end-to-end anastomosis to prevent anastomotic stricture/stenosis.

■ END-TO-END ANASTOMOSIS

Conceptually, the simplest anastomosis is the perpendicular, end-to-end anastomosis, depicted in **Figures 2A to C**. Corner sutures are placed 180° apart and are sewn toward each other in an over-and-over fashion. An end-to-end anastomosis can be employed when both ends of the vessel have adequate mobility, for example, in the case of trauma in which primary repair of the vessel can be done just by mobilizing the vessel/vein interposition grafting.

Technique of oblique end-to-end anastomosis to prevent anastomotic stricture/stenosis **(Figs. 3A to D)**.

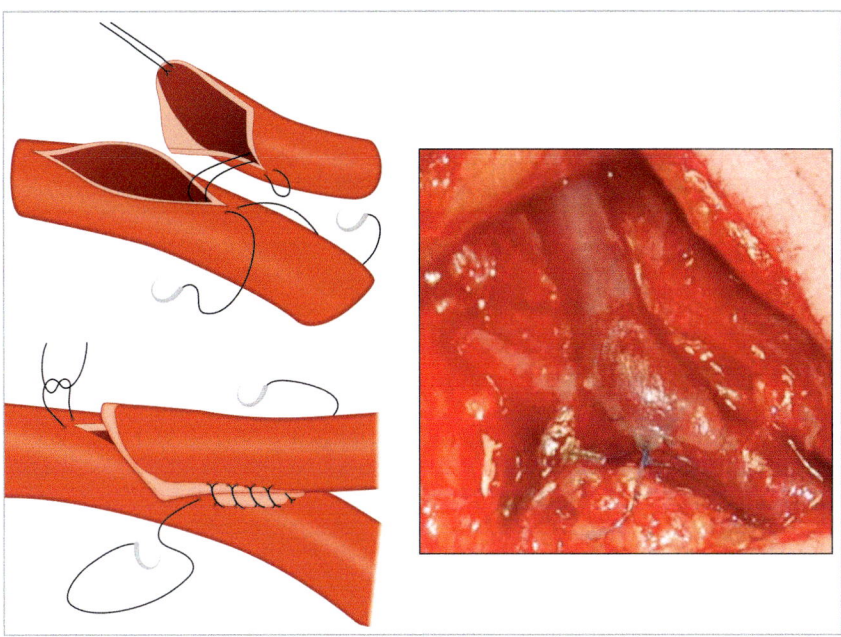

Fig. 4: Technique of end-to-side anastomosis.

This technique is rarely used because of the following drawbacks:
- The ends of the two vessels must have a fair amount of mobility to allow for easy and accurate placement of the sutures.
- This type of anastomosis tends to be constrictive if a running suture is used and drawn up tightly.

■ END-TO-SIDE ANASTOMOSIS

This is the most common prototype employed in arterial reconstructive surgery and is the basis of most bypass grafting which in principle attempts to provide a normal-caliber conduit for blood to flow around the diseased segment **(Fig. 4)**. An end-to-side anastomosis is used mainly in occlusive disease and the creation of an arteriovenous fistula.

One of the advantage of the technique is that it allows one to work with normal, or at least less diseased, vessels above and below the lesion, and to approach them at a convenient, accessible and familiar sites of exposure. When one uses the end-to-side anastomotic configuration, even remote bypass preserves pulsatile flow into each end of the bypassed segment. In comparison with bypasses with end-to-end anastomoses, one is no worse off hemodynamically if the bypass occludes. Further, one is better off in the event of infection, as the removal of the graft and closure of the suture line (usually with autogenous patch angioplasty) usually restore flow to the preoperative levels.

Depending on its diameter, the end of one vessel or, most commonly, the graft is either beveled at 30" (for larger vessels) or slit along one side with the corners trimmed (for smaller

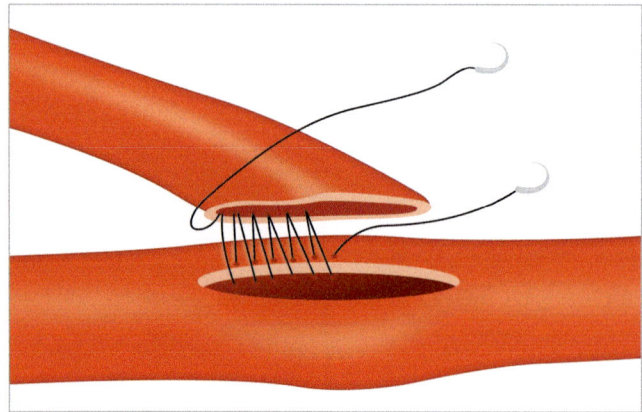

Fig. 5: Parachute technique.

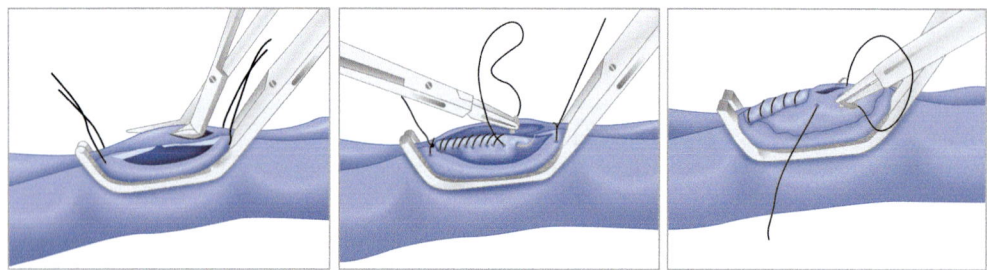

Fig. 6: Technique of side-to-side anastomosis between two large veins (e.g., portal and caval).

vessels). A longitudinal arteriotomy is then made in the side of the recipient vessel to match the slit in the longitudinal dimension. The anastomosis is begun with a horizontal mattress suture at the upper end of the cut end, or "heel," and continued along each side for about one-third of the way toward the middle. Then the tip, or "toe," of the graft is secured into the other corner of the recipient vessel with another mattress suture. The anastomosis is completed with a running suture that goes back along each side to meet its partner, to which it is tied.

Another approach, the "parachute technique," is useful in end-to-side anastomoses when the angle of entry is closer to perpendicular than usual and there is limited access to the far side of the anastomosis **(Fig. 5)**. The suture line is begun in the middle of the posterior aspect and simply run around either edge to the corner, before completing the anterior aspect of the anastomosis in the usual fashion.

■ SIDE-TO-SIDE ANASTOMOSIS

The side-to-side anastomosis is no longer commonly performed in clinical vascular surgery. The best known examples of this technique are probably the side-to-side portacaval shunt, Potts aortopulmonary anastomosis and Waterston aortopulmonary anastomosis **(Fig. 6)**.

24 How to Send a Sample for Biopsy?

Sunita Bhalla

■ INTRODUCTION

It is extremely important for the surgical residents to know a few basic facts about the field of histopathology and how samples from the operation theater complex are to be sent. Knowledge about this field will help you to ensure that the samples are well-preserved and sent in the appropriate solutions and containers for analysis. This chapter deals with the nitty-gritty of sending samples for histopathological examination.

Histopathology refers to the microscopic examination of the tissues removed as biopsies and resected specimens for the diagnosis and management of diseases including some autoimmune disorders. Broad-spectrum immunohistochemical, immunofluorescence, histochemical, and when needed ultrastructural techniques are used to identify abnormalities and disease processes precisely.

The tests performed are discussed here.

■ DIAGNOSTICS

- *Routine histopathology and immunohistochemistry*: These tests are conducted for the diagnosis of biopsies and resection specimens.
- *Frozen section*: This is a rapid procedure used to give intraoperative reports (within 10–15 minutes) on tissues to help the surgeon take critical decisions regarding patient management. It is used for diagnosis (benign/malignant), evaluation of margin status, assessing the adequacy of the sample, identifying the tissue sampled (for example, parathyroid tissue, nerves, and ganglion cells).
- *Microwave processing for urgent biopsies*: If a critical treatment decision is to be made on small biopsy diagnosis, a report can be given within 24 hours.
- *Histochemistry*: Histochemical stains such as Ziehl–Neelsen (ZN) stain for *Mycobacterium*, periodic acid-Schiff (PAS) stain for blood vessels, basement membrane, and fungus and silver stain for liver and kidney, and the fungus are used for the diagnostic purposes.
- *Immunohistochemistry*: An extensive panel of >110 antibodies is available to facilitate tumor differentiation and categorization.
- *Immunofluorescence*: Immunological disorders are diagnosed by using a panel of antibodies, including immunoglobulin G (IgG), immunoglobulin A (IgA), immunoglobulin M (IgM), C3, C1q, fibrin, kappa and lambda light chains to examine all kidney biopsies and some skin biopsies for classifying the renal and some skin disorders. Direct autoantibodies

tests such as anti-nuclear antibodies (ANA), anti-smooth muscle antibody (ASMA), antimitochondrial antibody test (AMA), anti-double stranded deoxyribonucleic acid (anti-dsDNA), antineutrophil cytoplasmic autoantibodies (ANCA), and phospholipase A2 receptor (PLA2R) are done by IF direct immunofluorescence.

The antiliver-kidney microsomal antibody (ALKMA) test is done by the line immunoassay (LIA).

Sample for Histopathology and Immunohistochemistry

You must take the following steps while collecting the sample:

- Transfer the specimen into the appropriate fixative immediately to prevent it from drying. This is especially important for small biopsies.
- The most commonly used fixative is 10% neutral buffered formalin, which you can procure from the department of pathology
- Bouin's fluid is preferred for testicular biopsies.
- The minimum amount of fixative that you should use is about ten times the size of the biopsy.
- You must immerse resection specimens completely in formalin soon after resection.
- Preferably avoid cutting open a specimen for better orientation.
- Make sure that the request form mentions the relevant clinical details and the type of surgery (excision or incision biopsy, core needle biopsy, resected specimen, or radical surgery). It must also include past history and previous biopsies conducted. Mention the previous biopsy number if it was conducted in this hospital, as well as the results of other laboratory and radiological investigations for correlation in the pathology department.

Mention what is specially required (for example, margins, any specific area for tumor infiltration, including specific blood vessels) in the request form. Label the margins of the specimen with sutures and specify this in the request form. Mention the contact number of the referring consultant/assisting resident in the request form so that he/she may be contacted for discussion if necessary. Indicate the clinical diagnosis for better evaluation of the tissue.

- Make sure that there is a bar code sticker with the patient's details on the request form and the container of the specimen to avoid mix-ups.
- Biohazardous samples, for example, those of patients with hepatitis B, C, human immunodeficiency virus (HIV) or tuberculosis, must have a warning sticker.
- In case of more than one sample from a patient, mention the site for each on the request form and the container.
- Microwave processing is done for quicker results. To ensure that the report is available on the same day, the biopsy must be sent before 12 noon to the histopathology department. Only small biopsies can be processed this way at the present.
- Specimens for frozen section must be fresh. Do not send them with any fixative. The request form must have the relevant clinical details and mention the type of surgery done. It must have the OT/contact number for conveying the report. Inform the pathologist about the requirement for frozen section.

- Immunohistochemistry (IHC) examination is conducted on tissue fixed in formalin, as in the case of routine histopathological examination. Please inform the patient that payment for IHC is to be made separately, apart from routine histopathology charges.
- Renal and skin biopsies for immunofluorescence must be sent in normal saline. Serum samples are required for autoantibodies tests and LIA.

PROTOCOL FOR REPORTING

- Reports for non-neoplastic lesions and benign tumors are made under the following heads:
  - Gross examination
  - Microscopic examination
  - Special stain interpretation (if done)
  - Immunohistochemical markers interpretation (if done)
  - Final diagnosis
- Cancer Protocol Templates (CAP) guidelines are followed for malignant cases. Tumor, node, and metastasis (TNM) staging is done.

  Special expertise is available on diseases of the female genital tract, gastrointestinal tract, brain and nerves, kidneys, heart and blood vessels, bones, skin, endocrines, soft tissues, including medical and surgical related diseases, and all forms of cancer and other tumors.
- Reports of frozen sections are conveyed to the clinician in the operating room telephonically. The written report has to be collected by the clinician/attendant from the reception.

CONCLUSION

The submission of a properly taken and well-preserved sample is important for a good pathologic evaluation. A properly written clinical history in the form is also of paramount importance to reach a good diagnosis. Good communication between the surgeon and the pathologist reporting the biopsy sample can not be underestimated.

25

Sample Collection in Microbiology

Sanghamitra Datta, Chand Wattal

■ INTRODUCTION

It is of paramount importance to know how a sample should be collected for microbiological examination as the quality of the report is directly proportional to the quality of the specimen processed. First and foremost, consider all samples as biohazardous and ensure that the universal precaution guidelines are followed during the collection and transport of the sample.

Factors affecting the quality of the specimen:

- Stringent practices should be followed, especially if the specimen is to be sent for culture sensitivity. Always inform the laboratory in advance if special handling of the sample is required.
- The consequences of a poorly collected and/or poorly transported specimen include failure to isolate the causative microorganism and recovery of contaminants or normal microbiota, which can lead to inappropriate treatment of the patient.
- Ideally, specimens should be collected before the administration of antimicrobial agents.
- The label on the container of the sample and the request form should not only mention the correct name of the patient and the date and time of collection, but also the type of sample and the source or site of collection. For example, if a pus sample from an abscess is sent, then the abscess site should be mentioned for better evaluation.
- All specimens should be transported to the laboratory promptly.

Samples for aerobic cultures and other microbiological tests are described here.

■ BLOOD

Sample Collection

Proper handwashing is the first requirement. You may use a hand rub instead. Wear gloves after drying your hands. Cleanse the selected venipuncture site with chlorhexidine [0.5% weight/volume (w/v) or 2.5% volume/volume (v/v)] in 70% alcohol. Wipe the site twice with the swab, concentrically from the center to the periphery, before pricking the vein. Do not palpate the vein after disinfecting the skin prior to inserting the needle.

Blood Culture

The number and timing of blood cultures is very important for an optimum yield of bacteria. A single sample may miss intermittent bacteremia and may cause diagnostic dilemmas in interpreting the clinical significance of certain organisms isolated. Hence, there is a need to conduct two or more blood cultures.

The following are recommended:

- *Acute sepsis*: Two samples from two sites before the initiation of antibiotic therapy.
- *Acute endocarditis*: Three to six blood cultures conducted with samples collected from three separate venipunctures over a period of 30 minutes to 1 hour.
- *Subacute endocarditis*: Three sets on day 1 (15 minutes or more apart), if all are negative, repeat after 24 hours.
- *Fever of unknown origin*: Two separate blood cultures at least 1 hour apart; if negative repeat after 24–48 hours.

Volume of Sample

- *Infants*: 0.5–1 mL
- *Children*: 1–10 mL
- *Adults*: 10–25 mL

Cerebrospinal Fluid

The fluid must be collected aseptically in sterile leak-proof tubes. Three samples are generally required for microbiology, hematology, and biochemistry testing. The second sample should be sent to the microbiology laboratory. The suggested volume is 5 mL for routine, fungal, and mycobacterial cultures for adults and can be lower for pediatric patients.

Other Sterile Body Fluids

Percutaneous aspiration of pleural, pericardial, peritoneal, and synovial fluids should be done aseptically. Air bubbles should be expelled from the syringe and the fluid must be stored immediately in a sterile screw-capped container or vial. Always submit as much fluid as possible. Never submit swab dipped in fluid.

■ URINE

Midstream urine needs to be collected as soon as the symptoms appear and ideally, prior to the initiation of antimicrobial therapy. The sample should never be collected from a bedpan or catheter bag.

- The urethral opening should be cleaned with water prior to collection to ensure that there is no contamination by the resident flora of the genital tract and clean catch urine should be collected in a sterile container.
- *Indwelling catheter sample*: The catheter collection port should be cleaned with 70% alcohol and punctured with a needle and syringe. The aspirated urine must be drained into a sterile container and sent to the laboratory as soon as possible.
  Collection of a specific urine pathogen and specimen type is shown in **Table 1**.

TABLE 1: Specific urine pathogens and specimen types.

Organism	Volume	Specimen type
Mycobacteria	>20 mL	First whole morning sample on 3 consecutive days; do not collect a 24-hour specimen

■ STOOL

Note the following points related to the collection of the sample:

- Stool may be passed directly into a wide-mouthed, leak-proof container with a tight-fitting lid.
- If it is passed in a clean, dry bedpan, it must be transferred into a sterile screw-capped container with a spatula.
- Keep the sample cool and do not incubate.
- Send stool for ova and parasites to the laboratory immediately after collection.
- If you use a rectal swab, pass the tip of the swab 1″ beyond the anal sphincter. Rotate the swab to sample the anal crypts and withdraw and place it in the transport media.
- All specimens should be sent to the laboratory within 30 minutes of collection.

■ SPECIMENS AND SAMPLES

Respiratory Tract Specimens

- Only designated Dacron or rayon swabs with plastic shafts should be used for oropharyngeal and nasopharyngeal specimens.
- Calcium alginate swabs or swabs with wooden sticks should not be used as they contain substances that inactivate some viruses and are inhibitory to the molecular assay.
- For oropharyngeal specimens, the swab should be inserted into the posterior pharynx and tonsillar areas without touching the tongue, teeth, and gums.
- For nasopharyngeal specimens, the swab should be inserted through the nares parallel to the palate and gently rolled to absorb secretions before removing.
- Swabs should be inserted into a sterile, designated vial with viral transport media. The tip of the applicator should be cut off to permit tightening of the cap of the tube.
- For expectorated sputum, the patient should rinse their mouth and gargle with water prior to sputum collection. The patient must not expectorate saliva or postnasal discharge into the container. To test for *Mycobacterium*, deeply coughed out sample must be collected on 3 consecutive days.
- Induced sputum using hypertonic saline vaporization is collected when the patient is unable to produce sputum on their own.
- For tracheostomy and endotracheal aspirations, the clinician should aspirate the specimen into a sterile sputum trap. Tracheostomy tube tip or endotracheal tube tip are not accepted.
- Bronchoscopy specimens include bronchoalveolar lavage, bronchial washing, bronchial brushing, and transbronchial biopsy specimens collected by clinicians and sent to the laboratory in screw-capped sterile containers.

Samples for Fungal Culture

Most specimens are collected in the same manner as specimens for bacteriological culture. Some specimens used solely for fungal testing should be collected in the following manner:

- *Hair*: Pluck out hair by the root with sterile forceps. Choose hairs that are broken and scaly and submit the specimen in a sterile Petri dish for processing and transport to the laboratory.
- *Nails*: Clean with 70% alcohol and scrape off the outer layers of the nail with a sterile blade. Scrape bits of the inner infected nail into a sterile Petri dish and transport to the laboratory.
- *Skin*: Clean with 70% alcohol to remove surface contaminants and scrape the outer portions of the red ring with a sterile scalpel. If there is no ring, scrape the area that looks most infected. Place the scrapings in a sterile Petri dish and transport to the laboratory.

Specimen for Anaerobic Culture

It is mandatory to consult the microbiologist on the transport medium and collection procedures. Aspirate the purulent material from the depth of the wound or abscess. Superficial material collected with a swab is not acceptable.

■ CONCLUSION

Technique of collection of samples for microbiology testing is important because errors may require the collection of new specimens, which may not be practical and may result in delay of appropriate treatment. Documentation and proper patient preparation are equally critical.

■ SUGGESTED READING

1. Baron EJ, Miller JM, Weinstein MP, Richter SS, Gilligan PH, Thomson RB Jr, et al. A guide to utilization of the microbiology laboratory for diagnosis of infectious diseases: 2013 recommendations by the Infectious Diseases Society of America (IDSA) and the American Society for Microbiology (ASM) (a). Clin Infect Dis. 2013;57(4):e22-121.
2. Falagas ME, Vergidis PI. Urinary tract infections in patients with urinary diversion. Am J Kidney Dis. 2005;46(6):1030-7.
3. Isenberg HD. Clinical Microbiology Procedures Handbook, 2nd edition. Washington DC: American Society for Microbiology; 2007.

CHAPTER 26

Use of Ultrasound in the Operation Theater: Vascular and Non-vascular Uses

K K Saxena

■ INTRODUCTION

David Robinson, a pioneer in ultrasonic imaging, first used the technique to see a live fetus way back in 1972. Multiple advancements were introduced in ultrasound technology after that. Probes (transducers) became smaller, the weight of the machine decreased and the resolution of the image improved. There was a switch from analog to digital systems and from cathode-ray tube (CRT) monitors to flat panel monitors. Intraoperative ultrasonic imaging was used for the first time in 1979 for the evaluation of biliary calculi.

Advances in medical technology have resulted in a higher rate of utilization of ultrasonic imaging in various intra-abdominal and vascular surgical procedures and in interventional procedures. Real time imaging of the organ of interest, characterization of any lesion and accurate localization has established the role of intraoperative ultrasonography (IOUS) in a large number of surgical procedures such as hepatic lobar resection, hepatic metastasectomy, renal surgery, breast surgery, partial pancreatectomy, and even some brain surgeries.

There are multiple indications for IOUS. These include localization of lesions, assistance in determining lesion resectability, clarifying indeterminate findings, and looking for multifocal lesions, liver transplant, kidney transplant, intraoperative guidance, intraoperative characterization for determining lesions and accurate planning of surgery, tumor staging, and metastatic survey. This chapter provides information about the use of IOUS in this institution.

■ EQUIPMENT AND TECHNIQUE

Various types of ultrasound machines are available with different types of transducers. Mostly transducers of high frequency (5–20 MHz) are used. The machines used are of G.E., Samsung, Philips, and Siemens. The probes are of different shapes. Convex array transducers with color Doppler and pulsed Doppler capabilities and volume are preferred. These probes may be T-shaped, linear, curvilinear, or hockey-shaped.

The probes are small and fit comfortably between the index and middle fingers of the operator, which allows the target organ to be palpated and scanned easily. Very good resolution of the superficial structures is needed for good localization of lesions.

The radiologist is a full member of the operating team, and must be scrubbed and dressed like a surgeon as per the institutional policy. He/she must ensure that there is sufficient space for examination. During examination, the light in the room should be as dim as possible and the monitor should be placed at such place/level that it can be seen easily.

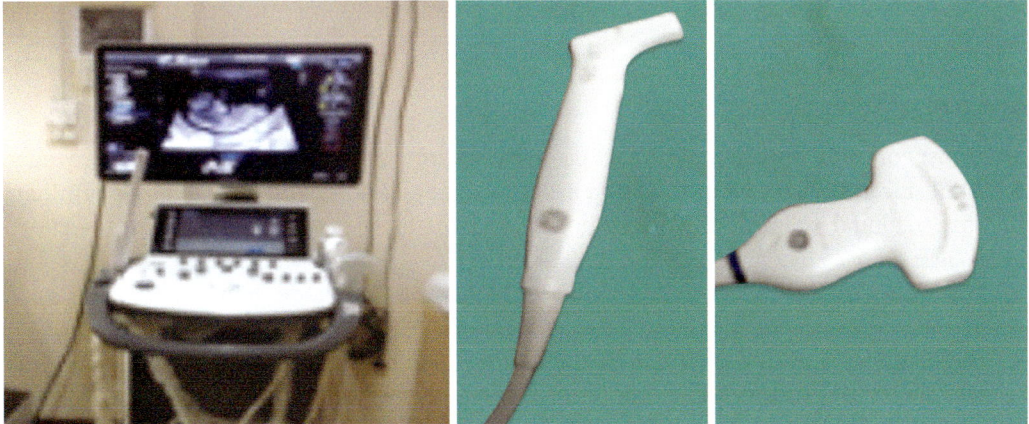

Fig. 1: High-end ultrasound machine, hockey stick (8–18 MHz), and convex probes.

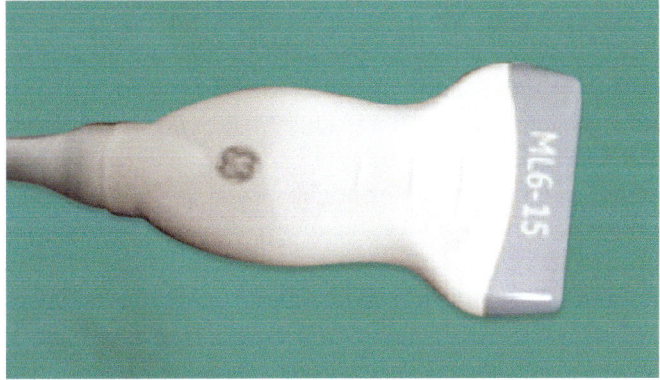

Fig. 2: High-resolution linear ultrasound probe (6–15 MHz) with color Doppler capabilities.

High-end ultrasound machine, hockey stick (8–18 MHz), and convex probes are depicted in **Figure 1**.

Transducers are sterilized by many methods. The best is to have a sterile membrane or sheath, which must be long enough to cover the electrical supply cord. Ethylene oxide gas may be used to sterilize the probe and supply cord, but this procedure takes long and may damage the contact area of the probe in the long run. The low-temperature hydrogen peroxide gas plasma technique has been introduced recently. This allows for the sterilization cycle to be completed in 2–3 hours and is safe to be used with heat sensitive probes. It enables the use of sterile transducers without a sheath or a condom. The liquid sterilization method is mostly not accepted by the surgeons because of inflammatory reactions. When using the sheath technique, use sterile gel to avoid the accidental puncture of the sheath and creating the problem of nonsterilized material. Sterile lukewarm isotonic saline is used for coupling between the sheath and the organ to be scanned.

High-resolution linear ultrasound probe (6–15 MHz) with color Doppler capabilities is depicted in **Figure 2**.

Coordination between the surgeon and the radiologist is very important to reduce the waiting time of the radiologist, who sometime feels that his/her time has been wasted.

■ APPLICATIONS

The most common application of IOUS is in liver surgeries such as segmentectomy, wedge resection, localization of metastasis, and liver transplant. Lesions which remain indeterminate in cross-sectional imaging may be evaluated by on the table core biopsy and frozen sections analysis.

- The spread of hepatocellular carcinomas into the walls of hepatic veins and bile ducts can be seen very easily by IOUS and helps in the staging of the tumor.
- Gallbladder status and calculi in the biliary duct and common bile duct can be seen very clearly by IOUS and decisions can be taken instantly for further action.
- Ultrasonic imaging plays a crucial role in conducting the transjugular intrahepatic portosystemic shunt (TIPS) procedure and is a major help for the interventional radiologist.
- Pancreatic tumors can be localized exactly during surgery. This is especially true of insulinomas before resection.
- Fibroids of the uterus can be localized exactly during surgery and may be ablated by cryosurgery under IOUS guidance.
- During surgery for the removal of breast lesions, IOUS is of great help to the surgeon for the exact retrieval of fine lesions.
- Small tumors of the kidney, which may not be picked up by routine ultrasound imaging, are best seen on IOUS, which provides guidance to the surgeon on the part to be resected.
- Brain screening can be conducted in the case of craniotomy or through burr holes. In infants, IOUS through the fontanelles can provide a lot of information. Tumors of the spinal cord can be localized precisely after laminectomy and using saline-filled area and IOUS.
- Small gastrinomas can also be seen by IOUS when there is a difficulty in localization during surgery.
- Biopsies must always be done under the OUS guidance to avoid accidentally puncturing an aneurysm with thrombus and prevent disaster.
- In carotid artery surgeries, IOUS has an important role in determining the presurgical and postsurgical status of the patency and reduction of the lumen of the vessels. Postprocedure clot formation may be checked immediately and measures may be taken accordingly. Doppler with biphasic and triphasic capabilities helps recognize normal or altered flows such as turbulence or stenotic flows by means of audible sounds too.
- Poststenting, the distal portion of the vessel can be judged immediately for good flow.

■ LIMITATIONS

This is a user-dependent modality and the radiologist needs a lot of experience to assess and provide the required information instantly. Some other factors involved are:

- Thickness of the patient
- Echogenicity of the patient
- Easy of approach to the organ
- Subjectivity

■ CONCLUSION

Though there has been a tremendous advancement in preoperative imaging of the liver, kidneys, pancreas, and vessels with multidetector computed tomography (MDCT), magnetic resonance imaging (MRI), and digital subtraction angiography (DSA), IOUS still provides important diagnostic information during surgery to help change surgical planning and patient management.

■ SUGGESTED READING

1. Choyke PL, Pavlovich CP, Daryanani KD, Hewitt SM, Linehan WM, Walther MM. Intraoperative ultrasound during renal parenchymal sparing surgery for hereditary renal cancers: a 10-year experience. J Urol. 2001;165(2):397-400.
2. Hellenthal NJ, Mansour AM, Hayn MH, Schwaab T. Is there a role for partial nephrectomy in patients with metastatic renal cell carcinoma? Urol Oncol. 2013; 31(1):36-41.
3. Kruskal JB, Kane RA. Intraoperative US of the liver: Techniques and clinical applications. Radiographics. 2006;26(4):1067-84.
4. Makuuchi M, Torzilli G, Machi J. History of intraoperative ultrasound. Ultrasound Med Biol. 1998;24(9):1229-42.
5. Marcal LP, Patnana M, Bhosale P, Bedi DG. Intraoperative abdominal ultrasound in oncologic imaging. World J Radiol. 2013;5(3): 51-60.
6. Plainfossé MC, Merran S. Work in progress: Intraoperative abdominal ultrasound. Radiology. 1983;147(3):829-32.
7. Sun MR, Brennan DD, Kruskal JB, Kane RA. Intraoperative ultrasonography of the pancreas. Radiographics. 2010;30(7):1935-53.

Surgeon and Surgical Instruments

R Sarangi

■ INTRODUCTION

Surgical instruments play a vital role in ensuring that surgical procedures are performed safely and in a manner that is convenient for the surgeon. In addition, they are designed to minimize the physical and mental strain on the surgeon. The earliest surgical procedures, performed in the Stone Age, were circumcision and trephination (making a hole) in the skull. Surgical procedures were performed in Mesopotamia as far back as 3,000 BC and in Babylonia in 1,700 BC. The instruments used were mostly sharp and pointed. It is recorded that in 2,500 BC, Egyptians used sharp instruments primarily to remove the brain from the body prior to mummification. The *Sushruta Samhita*, however, mentions the use of 20 sharp and 101 blunt surgical instruments. Galen (AD 130–200) gave a scientific narration on the appropriate use of surgical instruments. The modern era saw a dramatic change with the introduction of anesthesia and the pioneering work of Louis Pasteur (1822–1895) in microbiology in the mid-1800s that led up to antiseptic surgery.

■ CLASSIFICATION OF SURGICAL INSTRUMENTS

Surgical instruments are classified according to the objective for which they are used. They may be used for:
- Grasping tissue
- Cutting tissue
- Retracting tissue to facilitate the progress of the surgical procedure
- Controlling bleeding at the operation site (hemostat)
- Approximating tissue to close the operation wounds.

■ SURGICAL INSTRUMENTS

Various types of surgical instruments are used while performing different surgical procedures.

Scalpels, thumb forceps, artery forceps, retractors, scissors, needle holders, suction tubes, and dilators are the most commonly used instruments in day-to-day practice. These instruments assist the surgeon in performing the surgery comfortably.

The scalpel or lancet is the most basic surgical instrument and it is with the help of this that the surgeon starts the surgical procedure. It cuts the skin and underlying tissue at the operation site. Scalpels can be disposable or reusable. The blade attached to the tip of the instrument can be of different sizes. The surgeon selects the size according to the surgery he is performing. The scalpel can be used to perform simple surgical procedures such as incision and drainage of an abscess and cutting through the deeper structure in special circumstances.

Scissors, the other commonly used cutting instrument, are an important asset for the surgeon. They have a wide range of utility, starting from the simplest and most commonly performed action of cutting stitches to more complicated jobs such as cutting various types of body tissue, including fat, fibrous tissue, muscles, aponeurosis, and fascia. They are also used as a dissecting tool to create tissue planes.

Grasping forceps are meant to grasp the tissue on which the surgery is being performed. The tip may be fine or blunt, depending on the specific tissue being operated upon. Grasping forceps can be long or short, depending on the depth of the wound. Their basic purpose is to enable the surgeon to perform the procedure comfortably and meticulously. In special circumstances, the surgeon uses forceps with a specifically designed tip to prevent injury or damage to delicate organs such as blood vessels. Sometimes, the instrument is of help to the surgeon in holding tiny blood vessels to control bleeding. Subsequently, the surgeon seals the vessels with the help of cautery.

Clamps, too, are among the most commonly used instruments. They occlude vessels and other organs such as the bowel. They are designed differently to perform a particular function. Accordingly, they are known as traumatic or atraumatic. The atraumatic ones are used to hold the bowel or blood vessels, whereas the traumatic ones are used to hold bleeding vessels of less importance, subsequently to be ligated by suture or seals with the help of cautery. Clamps for occluding the bowel are specifically designed for the purpose and called *bowel clamps*. Similarly, those used to occlude blood vessels are called *vascular clamps*. The rest are known as hemostats.

Hemostats vary in size and shape. A hemostat can be straight or curved. It can be long or short, named as *mosquito forceps*. The long ones are used for deep operation wounds and the short ones for superficial wounds. Apart from the purposes for which forceps are usually used, they help the surgeon to hold the fascia and peritoneum capsule of an organ, and also to hold the stay sutures applied in special procedures on the bowel, bile duct, ureter, urinary bladder, etc.

A retractor is an extremely valuable instrument, adding as it does to the comfort of the surgeon, whether he is performing a simple or the most difficult operation. Simple in design, this instrument keeps unwanted structures or organs away from the operation field, thereby assisting the surgeon in performing the operation to his satisfaction. While small refractors are used to perform superficial surgical procedures, long, bladed, curved, or straight ones are used for procedures on deeper organs. These instruments are name after their inventors.

A needle driver or needle holder serves the function of closing the operation wound with sutures of various materials, depending on the structure or organ on which the surgeon is working. The size of the instrument depends directly on the site and the depth of the structure to be approximated or sutured. In addition, it depends on the size of the needle used to perform the procedure. In special circumstances, the needle holder is used to hold the needle and bring it out to the surface of the wound, in some special circumstances where with the assistant surgeon helping in doing this while the needle is still being held by the surgeon, after piercing through the tissue.

Suction tips and tubes play a vital role in keeping the surgical field free of blood or unwanted fluids. This helps the surgeon to visualize the anatomy of the operating field properly and carry out the procedure uneventfully. In special circumstances, these instruments also carry the irrigation fluid to cleanse the operating field and keep it dry so that the surgical procedure may continue smoothly.

Dilators and specula are basic surgical instruments used to access narrow passages and subsequent incisions to carry out the designated surgical procedure.

■ CONCLUSION

The right instrument for the right step makes surgery a smooth experience. Anticipation of the assistant and the OT scrub nurse as to the next step makes the job of the Surgeon a pleasant one and keeps the ambience of the operating theatre enjoyable and with good outcomes.

SECTION

3

Young Surgeon as the First Responder

CHAPTER 28

Anesthetist as the First Responder

Rashmi Jain

■ INTRODUCTION

During prehospital care of trauma patients, you must adopt a specific approach to their assessment and the treatment as this is important for their recovery. The control of catastrophic hemorrhage should be prioritized over the management of the airways and circulation issues. It is essential to address life-threatening and/or limb-threatening complications and immediately evacuate the person from the site of the accident to offer him/her definitive hospital care. Accidental injuries are an important cause of mortality and morbidity. Death is inevitable in the case of some catastrophic injuries and the person dies within a few minutes at the site of the accident. The causes of death can be classified into three broad categories:

- Airway obstruction, e.g., drowning and hanging, resulting in immediate death.
- Uncontrolled hemorrhage due to fractures, organ rupture, and vascular injuries, resulting in early death.
- Traumatic brain injuries, sepsis or multiorgan failure resulting in late death.

Emergency medical services focus on delivering definitive care within the first few hours (1–4 hours) of the traumatic incident. The concept of the "golden hour" refers to the need for such patients to receive early definitive care.

■ MASSIVE HEMORRHAGE

Mostly, bleeding from the extremities can be controlled by compression, elevation, and splinting with a cloth or bandage, which a first aid kit usually contains. This type of hemorrhage can be managed by the use of the mnemonic DDIT, which consists of the following steps. If one step fails, you must take the next.

- Use the dressing to apply direct pressure on the site of the bleeding.
- Superimpose another dressing to apply direct pressure.
- Apply indirect pressure by compressing the artery concerned against a bone.
- Apply a tourniquet if the bleeding is from a limb.

Suspected long bone fractures are reduced by splinting. A straight flat rod or stick can be tied to the limb to reduce the movement of the broken parts. Pelvic fractures are reduced by binding. A bandage or a long cloth can come in handy for this. Hemostatic agents can be applied to the site of the open wound. They are available in different forms, e.g., sprays or gauze impregnated with the agent. Patients with internal, noncompressible hemorrhage need to be transferred to the hospital immediately. Clinical ultrasonography can be done on the way to ascertain the site of bleeding. The clinical randomization of an antifibrinolytic in significant hemorrhage-2 (CRASH-2) trial has shown that intravenous tranexamic acid (an antifibrinolytic agent) is beneficial when administered within 3 hours of the occurrence of the injury.

■ AIRWAY/CERVICAL SPINE

The cervical spine should be stabilized in the event of an injury to the neck. The manual inline technique is used to achieve this, followed by the use of collars, blocks, scoops, or a vacuum mattress. The airway is managed concurrently with the stabilization of the cervical spine, after the hemorrhage has been controlled. There is no standardized practice for the airway management, which is a complex matter. In a patient with a reduced conscious level, airway patency can be achieved by the triple maneuver (jaw thrust, mouth open, and chin lift). Precautions should be taken in the case of patients with cervical spine injury. Debris can be removed from the mouth by a finger swipe or suctioning. Airway adjuncts such as the oropharyngeal airway or laryngeal mask airway (LMA), can be used for oxygenation and ventilation. In some cases, endotracheal intubation may be necessary to secure a definitive airway. These include patients with airway obstruction, ventilatory compromise, severe agitation and severe head injury. The first aid kits of all vehicles should be equipped with an AMBU bag and an LMA to secure the airway of patients. People should have a knowledge of basic life support. Driving licenses should be issued only if this basic requirement has been met.

■ BREATHING

A look, listen, and feel assessment of the patient's breathing will reveal if there is a life-threatening chest injury. Any open wound in the chest should be sealed immediately. A simple pneumothorax should not be treated. A tension pneumothorax causing ventilatory or hemodynamic compromise needs to be decompressed. In a spontaneously breathing patient, needle decompression should be followed by the insertion of a chest drain after he arrives at the hospital. A massive hemothorax should not be drained in the prehospital environment as this will cause a loss of the circulating volume of blood.

A patient with a severe head injury should benefit from intubation and ventilation, aimed at optimizing the cerebral perfusion pressure. These will improve oxygenation and prevent hypercarbia and hypoxia. Once airway patency has been established, high-flow oxygen therapy can be commenced. Patients with a head injury should be positioned head up, at 30°, and their endotracheal tube should be taped, and not tied to assist venous drainage from the head.

The patient's baseline neurological function should be assessed, using the "alert, voice, pain, and unresponsive (AVPU) scale" or the Glasgow Coma Scale. The size and reactivity of the pupils should be assessed. The patient's blood glucose level should also be checked as soon as possible.

Acute pain in trauma is undertreated and thus, leads to chronic pain issues. Ketamine is the drug of choice as it does not depress cardiovascular or laryngeal reflexes. The patient should be transferred to the hospital wrapped in such a way as to prevent further heat loss.

■ CIRCULATION

Early hemorrhage control should continue to be the area of focus to improve the outcome after road accidents. The degree of blood loss at the site of the accident can be assessed by heart rate, volume of the pulse, respiratory rate, and capillary refill time. Capillary refill time is an alternative to pulse rate, but is unreliable in the dark or in cold conditions. The amount of internal hemorrhage should be taken into account.

The treatment of blood loss begins with the establishment of intravenous lines (large bore) or an intraosseous line in the tibia. Ideally, first-aid kits should have intravenous fluids, cannulas and sets to start the administration of fluids. Current guidelines recommend minimum administration of cold and diluting crystalloid fluids in order to prevent hypothermia, coagulopathy, and acidosis.

The recommendations of the National Institute for Health and Care Excellence suggest volume resuscitation to achieve a palpable central pulse when the patient is shifted to the hospital. Ideally, blood products should be administered to make up for the blood loss. Blood warming devices are carried by emergency services in the developed countries. The guidelines of the Association of Anesthetists of Great Britain and Ireland advocate the provision of personnel who can administer anesthesia and carry out intubation in the prehospital phase. An alert should be sent to the destination hospital prior to the arrival so that it is better prepared to receive the trauma patient with blood products, an operation theater, etc. Standard operating procedures should be drawn up for prehospital trauma care to promote best practice and thus, improve outcomes.

Since the validation of the focused assessment with sonography for trauma (FAST) protocol, hand-held ultrasound devices are included in mobile intensive care units for out-of-hospital diagnosis performed by the emergency physicians. The French society of Emergency Medicine has recently issued its first national guidelines on emergency clinical ultrasonography (CUS). International recommendations now include CUS in cardiopulmonary resuscitation algorithms. Several randomized controlled studies are under way to evaluate the real contribution of CUS in the prehospital setting. The integration of CUS into the initial management of stable trauma patients will mark the end of plain film radiography.

■ CONCLUSION

From the point of view of cost-effectiveness, it is best to direct resources toward prehospital trauma services for the care of the injured and then toward hospital services for a better outcome. The emergency medical services of hospitals should work in partnership with the police department to play a proactive role in reducing trauma-related injury. Awareness programs should be conducted at the university level on the dangers of unsafe driving because the prevention of injuries obviates the need for treatment.

■ SUGGESTED READING

1. Bobbia X, Abou-Badra M, Hansel N, Pes P, Petrovic T, Claret PG, et al. Changes in the availability of bedside ultrasound practice in emergency rooms and prehospital settings in France. Anaesth Crit Care Pain Med. 2018;37(3):201-5.

2. Hamada SR, Delhaye N, Kerever S, Harrois A, Duranteau J. Integrating eFAST in the initial management of stable trauma patients: The end of plain film radiography. Ann Intensive Care. 2016;6:62.

3. Jørgensen H, Jensen CH, Dirks J. Does prehospital ultrasound improve treatment of the trauma patient? A systematic review. Eur J Emerg Med. 2010;17(5):249-53.

4. Krogh CL, Steinmetz J, Rudolph SS, Hesselfeldt R, Lippert FK, Berlac PA, et al. Effect of ultrasound training of physicians working in the prehospital setting. Scand J Trauma Resusc Emerg Med. 2016;24:99.

5. Lapostolle F, Petrovic T, Lenoir G, Catineau J, Galinski M, Metzger J, et al. Usefulness of hand-held ultrasound devices in out-of-hospital diagnosis performed by emergency physicians. Am J Emerg Med. 2006;24(2): 237-42.

6. Lockey DJ, Crewdson K, Davies G, Jenkins B, Klein J, Laird C, et al. AAGBI: Safer pre-hospital anaesthesia 2017: Association of Anaesthetists of Great Britain and Ireland. Anaesthesia. 2017;72(3):379-90.

7. Perel P, Al-Shahi Salman R, Kawahara T, Morris Z, Prieto-Merino D, Roberts I, et al. CRASH-2 (Clinical Randomisation of an Antifibrinolytic in Significant Haemorrhage) intracranial bleeding study: The effect of tranexamic acid in traumatic brain injury—a nested randomised, placebo-controlled trial. Health Technol Assess. 2012;16(13):iii-xii,1-54.

8. Rudolph SS, Sørensen MK, Svane C, Hesselfeldt R, Steinmetz J. Effect of prehospital ultrasound on clinical outcomes of non-trauma patients—a systematic review. Resuscitation. 2014;85(1):21-30.

9. Sadden F, Prior K. Anaesthetic priorities in pre-hospital trauma care. Anaesth Intensive Care Med. 2017;18(8):375-9.

29 Orthopedic Trauma

VK Nijhawan

■ INTRODUCTION

When Nicolas Andree coined the word "orthopedics," it referred mainly to the musculoskeletal "deformities." Little did he and his contemporaries know that one day, orthopedics would deal with almost every aspect of the musculoskeletal system, both "acute" conditions, as in "trauma," and "chronic" diseases of the bones and joints. Today, musculoskeletal trauma is an integral and important part of orthopedics. It is essential to assess and manage musculoskeletal injuries appropriately so as not to jeopardize life and limb. Orthopedic trauma care is especially concerned with the spine, pelvis, and extremities.

■ SPLINTING

The American College of Surgeons has laid down guidelines for life support in advanced trauma. The most important aspect of the management of an acute trauma event is splinting of the injured part. The technical use of simple devices is extremely valuable in this. You should avoid handling the injured part, whether it is necessary or unnecessary, unless it has been splinted. Splinting is important because if done properly, it helps control blood loss, reduces pain, prevents further soft tissue injury, facilitates the transportation of the patient and aids in the radiological assessment of the injury. If you are at the site of an accident, how do you manage the patient's injuries before he is transported to a medical center **(Fig. 1)**. How do you splint the injured part? You can use anything that is rigid as a splint, e.g., a walking stick or an umbrella. This can then be padded by something soft, such as a pillow. Folded magazines or newspapers make excellent splints for the arms or forearms. When everything else fails, bandaging the lower extremities together or fixing the arm in front of the torso helps. An injured leg or ankle can be bandaged with a pillow as the very bulk of the pillow helps

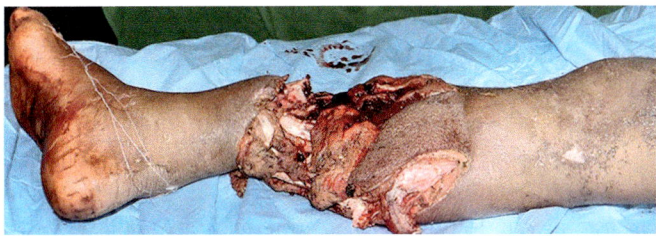

Fig. 1: Crush injury of foot.

to immobilize the area. Cramer wire splints, if available, are very useful for immobilization. They are like miniature ladders which can be bent into an appropriate shape, padded, and bandaged to the extremities. They do not interfere appreciably with the X-ray examination. Open fractures should be splinted the same way as closed fractures, except that the wound should be covered as early as possible. If sterile dressings are not available, covering the wound with even a clean handkerchief is better than not covering it at all. External bleeding is best managed by applying local pressure over the wound. The judicious use of a tourniquet may be useful and life-saving. After prehospital management, the patient should undergo the necessary radiographic examination and be managed further.

Polytrauma patients commonly present with collarbone fracture, either in isolation or associated with spinal trauma or thoracic trauma. The very weight of the arm is responsible for the excruciating pain in these cases. You can relieve the pain by folding any piece of cloth to make a triangular sling to support the weight of the arm. Such a sling can be used for a fracture of the shaft of the humerus as well.

■ SPINAL INJURY

Injury of the spine, with or without neurological deficit, must always be considered in patients with multiple injuries. About 55% of spinal injuries occur in the cervical region, 15% in the thoracic region, 15% at the thoracolumbar junction and 15% at the lumbosacral junction. You must remember that in cases of spinal trauma, excessive manipulation without adequate immobilization may cause additional neurological damage and worsen the patient's outcome. The general management of spinal trauma includes immobilization, intravenous fluids, and medications. The presence of paraplegia or quadriplegia is presumptive evidence of cervical spine instability. The presence of paraplegia or a level of sensory loss on the chest or abdomen is presumptive evidence of thoracolumbar instability. Immobilization plays a crucial role in the spinal trauma. In cervical spine injury, before and during the transfer of the patient to a definitive care facility, a semirigid cervical collar must be used for continuous immobilization of the entire body. In addition, the head should be immobilized with the help of a backboard, tape, and straps. Flexion and extension of the neck should be avoided. The airway is of critical importance in patients with spinal cord injury and early intubation is necessary if there is evidence of respiratory compromise. During intubation, the neck must be maintained in a neutral position.

■ PELVIC TRAUMA

Pelvic trauma is an emergency and warrants thorough evaluation from head to toe since it is associated with high-energy impact. It may present in isolation, but is mostly associated with trauma of either the head, thorax, abdomen, or extremities. Retroperitoneal bleeding is one of the worst aspects of pelvic trauma. You need to manage it temporally at the site of the accident by using any piece of cloth as a sling to facilitate immobilization. The sling acts like a binder which helps to stabilize the fracture fragments and hence, controls the bleeding. For injuries such as fractures of long bones, orthopedists have at their disposal a very useful splint, called the Thomas splint, which has saved the lives of thousands of victims. If available at the site of the injury, it can be used to alleviate pain and also, to help control bleeding. Further, transportation of the patient from the site of the accident becomes much easier once the Thomas splint is secured to the injured limb.

You must keep in mind that you can convert things which are conveniently and easily available into tools that can help to save the lives of trauma victims at the roadside. It could be a stick, a piece of cloth, a board of wood, cardboard, newspaper, or even an umbrella. Regular interaction with the public is a must to make people understand how these simple tools can be used as first aid to help save lives.

Superficial Injuries and Burns

R Khazanchi

■ INTRODUCTION

Plastic surgeons deal with a variety of injuries to different areas of the body. These include faciomaxillary injuries, hand injuries, skin avulsion injuries, and burns. I will briefly describe what you should do if you come across any of these injures at the site of an accident.

■ HAND INJURIES

The hand is a specialized organ, which requires special care when injured. At the site of an accident, the first thing that may scare you is the bleeding. The best way to control bleeding is to apply direct pressure and elevate the hand and arm. The use of a tourniquet should be avoided as far as possible and should be considered only in the last resort. Sometimes, there are cases in which an artery is partially divided and does not stop bleeding even after the application of direct pressure. You then have to apply a tourniquet proximal to the site of injury.

Splinting and relief of pain are the next most important features of the management of hand injuries. Use analgesics to relieve the pain. Splintage is important in injuries which cause a partial amputation. It helps to preserve the circulation to the partially amputated part. You should replace the part in the best possible anatomical position and then splint it with an improvised splint, such as a rolled up newspaper or magazine. In the case of a complete amputation, you must not only control bleeding from the stump, but also retrieve the amputated part and transport it in a specialized manner because the ultimate survival of the part depends on how well you preserve it. The best thing to do is to put it in a polythene bag, seal the bag by tying a knot on top of it and put the bag into another polythene bag filled with ice. It is important to make sure that the ice does not come in direct contact with the amputated part. In warm climates, if the patient and the amputated part have to be taken to a hospital that is far away, the bag should be transported in a thermocol box or a vacuum flask. It is important to ensure that water does not come in direct contact with the amputated part because being hypotonic, it gets absorbed into the vascular endothelium and compromises the ultimate survival of the part.

■ AVULSION INJURIES

Avulsion injuries of the skin may be partial, i.e., when the skin is still attached to the body, or complete, i.e., when the skin has separated from the body altogether. In partial avulsion, you should put the skin back where it should be and then apply whatever dressing is available. You could also wrap it in a towel and put a bandage over the towel. In cases in which the skin has avulsed completely, you must be very particular about not allowing structures such as tendons and nerves to dry. The best thing to do is to wrap the area in a wet towel and transport the patient to the hospital.

■ BURNS

In the case of thermal burns, remove the victim from the scene of the fire and roll him/her on the floor, wrap him/her in blankets or pour water to stop the clothes from burning. Once you have managed to do this, take off all the burnt clothes and pour copious amounts of tap water on the victim's body. There is a misconception that one should use cold water. Cold water can be harmful for patients with extensive burns because it may cause severe hypothermia. It is only for minor burns that you can use cold water. Also, once the patient's clothes are no longer aflame, make sure not to cover him/her with blankets. If you suspect inhalation injury, which happens when the victim is trapped in a fire in a closed space, administer oxygen as early as possible. Many lives could have been saved in the Uphaar case if this practice had been followed during transportation.

In the case of chemical burns, wash the affected area with copious amounts of tap water, regardless of whether the burn is caused by an acid or alkali. Using an opposite chemical (acidic or alkaline) would produce an exothermic reaction, which would make matters worse.

As for electrical burns, first switch off the electrical supply unit. The only immediate danger to a patient with electrical burns is the possibility of a cardiac complication or cardiac arrest, in which case cardiopulmonary resuscitation has to be instituted. And what should you do with the burn wound? We often get patients who have applied Burnol or used some home remedy, such as oil or ink. The best is not to apply anything because it interferes with the assessment of the depth of the burn. Cover the burn with a clean sheet or clean towel and transport the patient to a hospital.

31

Trauma and the Vascular Surgeon

Rajiv Parekh

■ INTRODUCTION

It is not possible to perform appropriate vascular surgery at the roadside, where specialized techniques cannot be used. There are not many things you can do if a patient is bleeding to death at the roadside. Essentially, what you need to know are a few tricks to help sustain the patient so that he/she can be shifted to a hospital. Apart from being familiar with the airway, breathing, and circulation (ABC) of cardiac resuscitation, it would be useful if you could locate a clinic or some small place which could provide some type of first aid before the patient is shifted to a hospital. If there is a hemorrhage for which ice is required and the patient is in shock, there is obviously no shortcut to the resuscitation. You must resuscitate the patient and try to control the bleeding to save his/her life.

Bleeding can be external or concealed. External bleeding is not easy to control if it is in the region of the neck or if there is an open wound, and thumb pressure fails to do the job. By and large, however, thumb pressure at the site of the injury can do wonders, if it is applied against a bone, since you cannot compress a vessel unless there is a hard structure behind it. If you compress an artery against a bone, you will achieve hemostasis. The neck is not the kind of place where you can tie a tourniquet. The management of bleeding in the limbs is slightly different because there is a lot that can be done to save a limb. First you can try thumb pressure. If this does not work, you can apply pressure with two fingers, and then palm pressure. If these methods do not succeed, seek the help of your assistant. If there is a big wound and you cannot compress the area, the spurter has to be tied off. In the movie Black Hawk Down, there is a young American soldier whose limb gets shot off. Some of the other soldiers try to compress the wound, but it does not work because the femoral artery has retracted into the pelvis. Since they do not have any help, they fish blindly into the wound with their bare hands. They can now feel the pulsating artery, and they pull it up and put a clamp across it. I narrate this because this is something which can be done, but obviously, you would need some sort of help at the roadside. You can use compression to stop bleeding even from the aorta. If you come across a case of bleeding ruptured aortic aneurysm, you can control the bleeding after a laparotomy and stabilize the patient by applying pressure on the infrarenal aorta, as the case may be. It is necessary for all the doctors to have a knowledge of the "regional safety zone," which means that you need to know the site of approach to achieve vascular control. You must make an approach through an area or zone which is safer to enter and which is far or as far as possible from the site of bleeding, at the same time, your point of approach should give you adequate control to ensure the safety of the limb, viscera, etc.

If you have been able to control the bleeding either with compression or a tourniquet, do not use the tourniquet indefinitely. If compression with the thumb or fist works, do not apply a tourniquet because it will do more damage. You can fashion a tourniquet out of just about anything, e.g., a tie, belt, piece of string or cloth. To tighten the tourniquet, you do not really need to tie a tight knot, as this will slip. All you need to do is to tighten it fast and rotate it. Then every turn will tighten the tourniquet, which is not possible if you tie a knot. It is essential to know how long the tourniquet should be used, because you might end up causing ischemia and gangrene without meaning to. You must keep in mind that a limb can survive up to 90 minutes of complete occlusion of the main arteries.

If there is a small cut over the radial artery or a small vein that is bleeding, the definitive procedure would be to find it and tie it. Merely getting hold of the spurting artery and tying it off—even if it is a major limb artery—may save a life, although the victim may lose a limb. Needless to say, it is best to have a live patient, who can be shifted to a place where the tied artery can be reconstituted. If the source of bleeding cannot be identified, you can always refer the patient to a hospital. You may have saved a life, which is a great achievement.

When dealing with bleeding from the carotid artery, your knowledge of anatomy should tell you that it runs across the front of the transverse processes of the 6th cervical vertebra. Thus, you can compress the common carotid, external carotid and internal carotid against the bone. Compressing it with the thumb works perfectly well. In a young patient who has suffered trauma, even if you occlude one of the common carotid arteries, it usually does not cause any problems unless, of course, there is a deficiency of the other common carotid artery, which is very rare. In the absence of this complication, you can go ahead and occlude it and keep it occluded. If you are in a small setup, then you will have to tie it. Go ahead and do so as nothing will go wrong.

If you can feel the carotid artery against the bone, you can compress it. Take note that the artery must be compressed against a bone, a hard structure behind it. The carotid is ideal for the purpose of compression since there is bone all along its course, and you can easily compress it across the 6th cervical vertebra.

32 Primary Management of Ocular Trauma in Polytrauma

AK Grover

■ INTRODUCTION

Patients of polytrauma often have associated eye injuries. These can range from minor disorders, such as subconjunctival hemorrhages and corneal abrasions, to severe forms, such as optic nerve avulsion and globe rupture leading to irreversible loss of vision. In polytrauma, systemic evaluation and management are given top priority. However, once the systemic assessment has been made, ocular examination should not be overlooked. Multiple structures may be involved in eye trauma. The management of globe injuries takes precedence over injuries involving the ocular adnexa (eyelids, lacrimal apparatus, and bony orbit).

Worldwide, around 1.6 million people become bilaterally blind, about 2.3 million become bilaterally visually impaired and 19 million suffer unilateral loss of vision due to ocular trauma. Visual loss due to ocular trauma has a profound socioeconomic impact, resulting in loss of productivity, and a need for care facilities and rehabilitation. The timing of the intervention is critical. In the management of chemical burns, every second is of extreme importance. Globe injuries should be repaired within hours. Lacrimal and eyelid lacerations should be repaired within a day or two, while orbital injuries can wait a week or two.

Immediate and adequate treatment of ocular trauma can make all the difference between retained vision and blindness. The primary management of eye injuries is based mainly on two factors:
1. The mechanisms of the injury
2. The structures of the eye involved

■ MECHANISMS OF THE INJURY

Injuries can occur by the following mechanisms:

Blunt Trauma

This results from an impact by a blunt object. The object may damage the internal structures of the eye, often leading to intraocular hemorrhage within the anterior chamber or posterior chamber, uveal injuries, lens injuries in the form of subluxation, dislocation or rupture, and retinal injuries and detachment. The force exerted by the blunt object can also cause rupture of the globe, with or without extrusion of the contents. It may also lead to lacerations of the eyelid or orbital fracture resulting in restriction of motility **(Fig. 1)**.

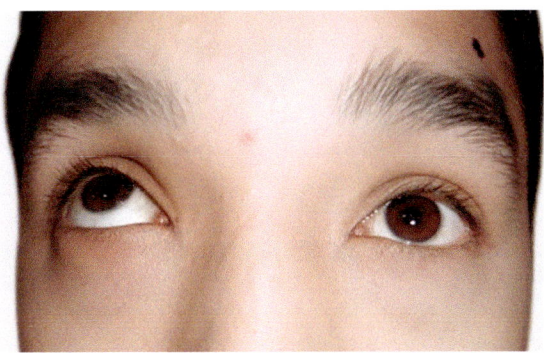

Fig. 1: Restriction of eye movements in a child after blunt trauma with fracture of the Orbital floor.

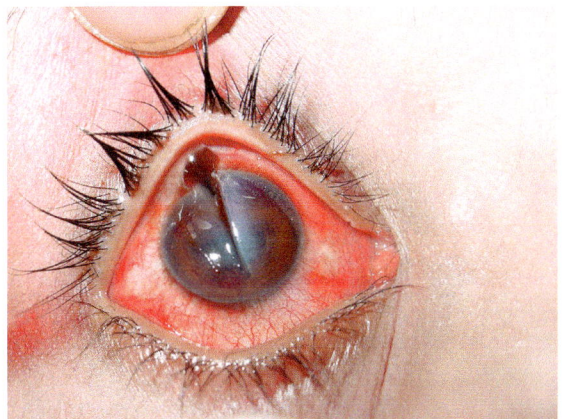

Fig. 2: Open globe injury caused by a sharp object.

Penetrating Trauma

This occurs when a sharp object pierces the external coats of the eyeball, such as the cornea or sclera. The laceration may be a full-thickness or partial-thickness injury **(Fig. 2)**. Projectiles, such as pieces of glass, shrapnel or pellets, which have enough velocity can penetrate the eye and get retained inside in the form of an intraocular foreign body.

Thermal and Chemical Burns

The former occur due to exposure to a hot or burning object and the latter due to exposure to chemicals, whether acidic or alkaline **(Fig. 3)**. The two types of exposure may even be combined, as in firecracker injuries or exposure to quick lime.

■ STRUCTURES OF THE EYE INVOLVED

The injury can involve one or multiple structures of the eye and orbit. Eyelid injuries can take the form of lacerations or tears **(Fig. 4)**. They may also involve the tear drainage apparatus

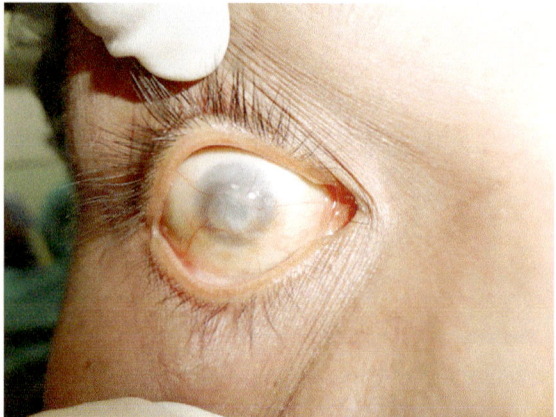
Fig. 3: Corneal opacity caused by a chemical injury.

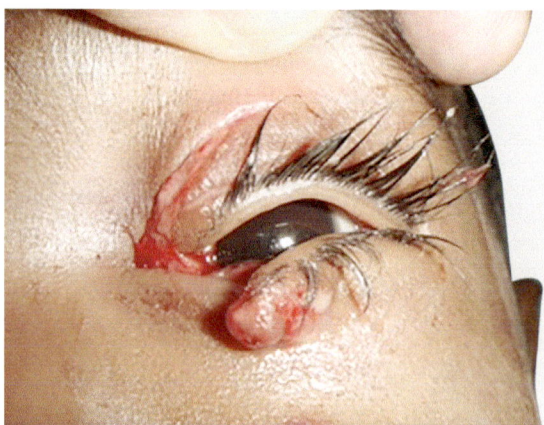
Fig. 4: Eyelid laceration and injury to canalicular (proximal part of tear duct) by a blunt trauma.

(lacrimal apparatus). As for the orbit, there may be an orbital wall fracture or orbital hemorrhage. In addition, there may be injuries to the orbital contents, such as the lacrimal gland, optic nerve, and ophthalmic vessels. The eyeball itself may be involved, alone or in association with other structures.

■ EXAMINATION

In all cases of suspected eye injury, you must elicit a proper history, whenever possible. It is necessary to carry out a visual acuity assessment by whatever method is practical under the circumstances, to determine whether the visual loss is mild or profound. You must also check for the presence of double vision, which indicates nerve, muscle, or bone injuries. You should examine the eyelids under torchlight to ascertain whether there are any injuries. Use a torch to examine the anterior segment, and check the size and reactions of the pupil. Make a note of any abnormality. Check for the presence of the fundal glow and its brightness, and compare it with the other eye, using an ophthalmoscope. This primary examination will give you an idea of the type of injury and its severity, which helps plan further management.

■ MANAGEMENT

Blunt Trauma

Vision of <6/12 in the affected eye or double vision suggests significant ocular injury. The presence of blood in the anterior chamber (hyphema) also suggests injury to the internal structures of the eye. You should note the reactions, size, and shape of the pupil. Any signs of globe rupture, such as a visible tear or laceration or the extrusion of intraocular contents, suggest severe eye injury and require prompt surgical intervention. The presence of any of the symptoms mentioned above warrants management by an ophthalmic surgeon.

Penetrating Trauma

Patients of penetrating trauma have a soft-looking eye, with distortion of the globe structures and protrusion of the black/brown uveal mass. The fundal glow is either absent or faint. You should take care not to put pressure on an already compromised eyeball, so cover it with a pad or shield for protection. Administer antibiotics and analgesics to the patient, who should be kept fasting. A preanesthetic check-up should be carried out before surgical intervention. You should order a CT scan (or if this is not available, an X-ray) of the orbit to detect any associated intraocular or orbital foreign bodies. This will also help to diagnose any associated orbital wall fractures. It is very important to be prompt in making a referral to an ophthalmologist and planning for surgical intervention, as the earlier you manage the injury, the better the results.

Chemical and Thermal Burns

Chemical burns are true ophthalmic emergencies. Alkali injuries are much more hazardous than acidic ones, as they cause saponification and penetrate deep into the ocular tissues. The first aid treatment of chemical burns should be carried out on the spot, and consists of immediate and copious irrigation of the eye with saline or any clean fluid, including tap water. This should be continued for at least 30 minutes or until the pH of the conjunctival sac is neutralized. You should meticulously remove any retained particles of chemical (as in lime burn) as they may continue to alter the pH. You must remember that each passing minute worsens the prognosis, so the treatment should be started without wasting any time.

In the cases of lacerations and tears of the eyelid, bleeding should be stopped primarily with a pressure bandage. You must rule out other ocular injuries. Administer antibiotics and analgesics and plan for repairs within the next 24–36 hours.

Orbital Fractures

Orbital fractures may be manifested as diplopia, proptosis, enophthalmos, ecchymosis, and displacement of the globe. The diagnosis can be confirmed by CT scan or X-ray of the orbit. Surgical repair is carried out once the inflammation and swelling subside.

■ CONCLUSIONS AND RECOMMENDATIONS

The early detection and diagnosis of eye injuries are essential for proper management and preservation of vision. When cases of polytrauma are brought to the emergency department, they are initially examined by the emergency doctor on duty and are managed primarily by a team of physicians, orthopedic surgeons, and anesthetists. It is, however, of vital importance to check for ocular injuries and to assess the nature and severity of such injuries in order to determine the need for further referral and management.

■ ACKNOWLEDGMENTS

Shaloo Bageja, Amrita Sawhney, and Harsh Rathod.

■ SUGGESTED READING

1. Boyd S, Sternberg P, Recchia F. Modern Management of Ocular Trauma. New Delhi: Jaypee Brothers Medical Publishers; 2009.
2. Kahana A. Orbital disease and surgery. In: Smith BC (Ed). Ophthalmic Plastic and Reconstructive Surgery. St. Louis: Mosby; 1987.
3. Kuhn F, Pieramici DJ. Ocular Trauma: Principles and Practice. New York: Thieme; 2002.

Roadside Trauma in a Pregnant Patient: The Obstetrician's Role

Harsha Khullar

■ INTRODUCTION

Cases of obstetric trauma are complex and require multidisciplinary care, both of the mother and unborn child. Obstetric trauma is a leading cause of nonobstetric mortality. Seven percent of pregnant women suffer trauma. Of these, >50% are due to motor vehicle accidents. Vehicular crashes are the most common cause of serious life-threatening trauma or blunt trauma to the fetus. Domestic abuse and assault account for 22.3% of the cases of trauma in obstetric patients, falls for 21.8%, and penetrating injuries for 1.3%. Trauma in obstetric patients poses a problem because the signs and symptoms may be altered due to the fact that one has to deal with two patients (mother and fetus). The treatment priorities are the same as in other cases of trauma, but you need to modify the resuscitation methods and management strategy to accommodate the physiological and anatomical changes caused by pregnancy.

The following are the anatomical changes you should keep in mind **(Fig. 1)**. In the first trimester, the uterus is thick-walled and intrapelvic. After 12 weeks, it comes out of the pelvis and becomes intra-abdominal. In the second trimester, the uterus contains a large amount of amniotic fluid. In the third, it is very thin-walled and the fetal head is large. At 36 weeks, the uterus reaches the costal margin. Finally, in the last 2–8 weeks, the fetal head descends to become engaged in the pelvis.

As fetal death is a consequence of the maternal death, the main guidelines for managing pregnant patients who have sustained trauma is to ensure maternal survival. Other than promptness, a skilled team approach is required, backed by a knowledge of the altered

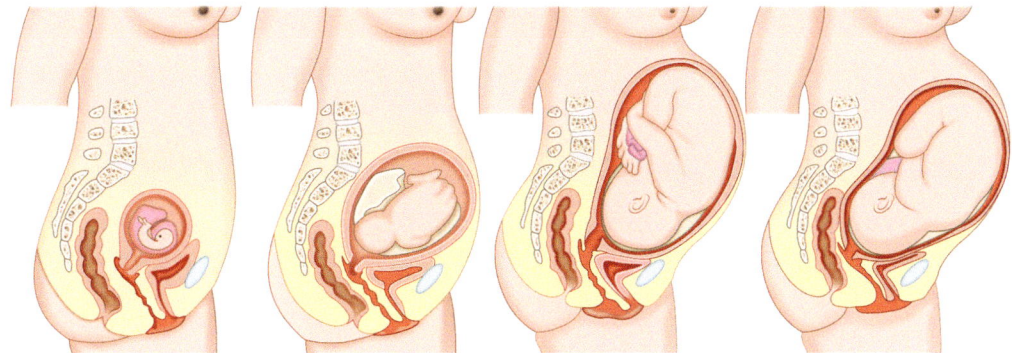

Fig. 1: Altered anatomy in pregnancy.

anatomical and physiological changes associated with pregnancy. It is important to note that of all pregnant patients who present with trauma, 11.4% go into preterm labor and 1.58% can present with abruptio placentae. The signs and symptoms of injury may also be altered due to the gravid uterus. Fetal demise may be due to maternal hypotension, maternal pelvic fracture or uterine rupture.

■ TYPES OF INJURY

There are two types of injury to consider in obstetric trauma—(1) blunt injury and (2) penetrating injury. In blunt injuries, as among accident victims, head injuries need to be ruled out. These injuries may be associated with retroperitoneal hemorrhage, abruptio placentae, or uterine rupture. Considering that 1–3% of pregnant women have been found to be involved in motor vehicle accidents, it is very important that they wear their seat belts properly. The seat belt should be as low as possible on the pregnancy bulge, across the anterior superior iliac spine and pubic symphysis **(Fig. 2)**. If the belt is placed on the uterus, the force transmitted to the uterus increases by 3–4 times. The shoulder harness should be positioned between the breasts.

Stab injuries are rare among pregnant patients. However, they are associated with a mortality rate of 93% and a morbidity rate of 50%. The gravid uterus alters the pattern of injury to the mother. The probability of harm increases if the weapon enters the upper abdomen. If it enters below the uterine fundus, maternal visceral injury is less likely, but the fetal death rate

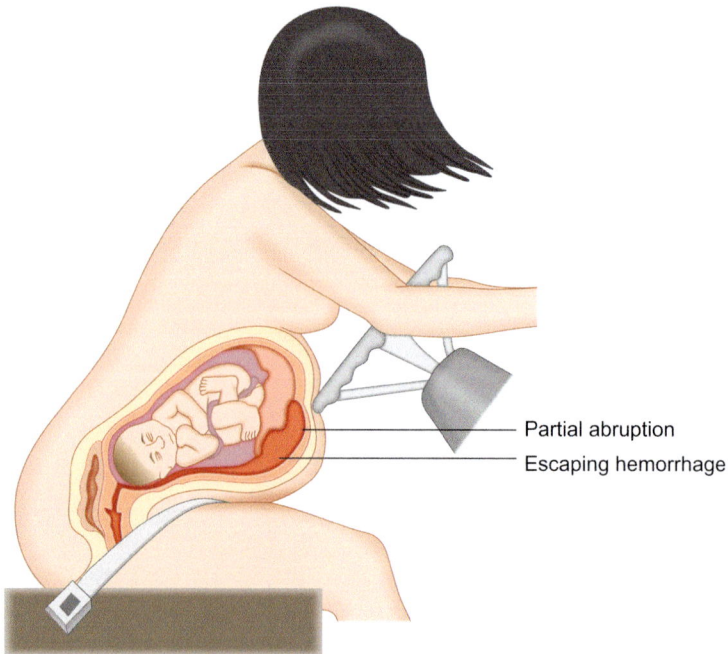

Partial abruption
Escaping hemorrhage

Fig. 2: Roadside trauma in pregnancy.

approaches 67%. However, the fetal death rate is 38% if the injury is above the uterus. Uterine rupture is more likely in the case of a previously scarred uterus.

You should not underestimate obstetric trauma caused by physical assault and abuse. You must always keep the possibility of domestic violence in mind, even though many patients are unwilling to talk about it to family and friends.

■ CONSEQUENCES OF INJURY

- *Premature contractions*: These rarely progresses to preterm delivery. Tocolysis has not been seen to have a proven advantage in cases of trauma.
- *Abruptio placentae*: This occurs due to differential elastic properties in the uterus and results in shearing of the placenta. It is associated with 3% of minor trauma and up to 50% of severe trauma cases.
- *Uterine rupture*: A rare complication, this occurs in 0.6% of cases of severe abdominal trauma. It results from direct trauma after 12 weeks of gestation. A history of prior surgery increases the risk.
- *Maternal fetal hemorrhage*: In the first trimester, the incidence is 3%, in the second 12%, and in the third 45%. Maternal fetal hemorrhage causes isoimmunization and fetal death. The Kleihauer–Betke test is used to assess fetomaternal hemorrhage although it may be impossible to carry out this test at the roadside.
- *Uterine rupture*: Less than 1% of severe cases of obstetric trauma result in uterine rupture due to blunt trauma. Uterine rupture is more likely to occur in cases in which the uterus has been previously scarred. It is usually associated with the direct impact of a substantive force. Decelerative force following a 25 mph collision can generate intrauterine pressure of up to 500 mm Hg in a woman using proper restraints. Various degrees of injury, ranging from serosal hemorrhage to complete avulsion, may occur. Seventy-five percent of cases involve the fundus. Maternal mortality from uterine rupture is 10%, though it is usually other associated injuries that cause death.
- *Fetomaternal hemorrhage*: The hemorrhage may either be small or massive. While 90% of cases fall in the first category (amount of blood <15 mL), in rare cases, the hemorrhage is massive.
- *Fetal injury and death*: Major vehicle crashes account for 82% of fetal deaths, which may result from maternal shock, pelvic fracture, maternal head injury and hypoxia. Fetal skull and brain injuries are common. They are more likely if the head is engaged in the maternal pelvis, on impact and if the head is unengaged or if it is a nonvertex presentation (fetal head injury from contrecoup effect).

The **ABC of the resuscitation** of pregnant victims of roadside trauma is the same as for other patients. "A" stands for airway assess and control, "B" denotes breathing, and "C" circulation. It is best if intravenous access if possible. When being transported, the patient should be placed in the **left lateral position**. The prehospitalization priorities include giving the patient oxygen (if available) by mask and anticipation of shock. Further, the expected date of delivery should be noted, if possible, by taking the patient's history.

■ MANAGEMENT

The management of pregnant women who have suffered trauma should be well coordinated and a multidisciplinary approach by skilled personnel is of paramount importance. The guiding principle should be that resuscitating the mother will resuscitate the fetus. The basic principles of management include the following:

- Be aggressive/temperate, using common sense
- Avoid obstruction and do not focus too much on the fetus
- An apparently stable mother may be compensating at the cost of the fetus
- If the woman is >24 weeks pregnant, a cardiotocography has to be done.

Four-minute Rule

Maternal cardiopulmonary resuscitation (CPR) should be carried out for 4 minutes. The infant should be delivered by the fifth minute for a good fetal outcome. If maternal CPR exceeds minutes, fetal survival is unlikely. The chance of survival is 0% at <23 weeks gestation.

Prevention of Traumatic Fetal Deaths

It is advisable that all pregnant women be educated and given prenatal counseling on their safety and the precautions they should take to avoid trauma. They must be advised to use seat belts and should be counseled on the proper use of air bags. Fetal mortality is thrice as high in the case of women who do not wear seat belts. A survey found that 86% of pregnant women used restraints, but 50% used them incorrectly. Three women in the third trimester whose driver side air bag deployed in 10–25 mph collision had no injuries. Placental abruption has been reported in up to 20% of women whose air bags deployed in collisions at a speed of 40 mph.

Associated Emotional Trauma

If a pregnant woman is in a highly fearful state, the fear gives rise to a metabolic cascade. Chronic anxiety can set the stage for a whole array of trauma based such as prematurity. The woman's neurotransmitters create a chemical and physical imprint on the baby's brain and body.

For Hemodynamically Unstable Mother

Resuscitation, followed by urgent transportation to the nearest medical facility, is of paramount importance. The following protocol can be followed once the patient reaches a medical center **(Flowchart 1)**.

■ POINTS TO REMEMBER

- Trauma during pregnancy contributes significantly to maternal and perinatal mortality and morbidity. The contribution of physical assault and abuse should not be underestimated.
- All Rh-negative pregnant women sustaining blunt trauma should receive anti-D immunoglobulin.
- All pregnant women should receive prenatal counseling and education on ways of ensuring their safety and the precautions required to avoid trauma.

Flowchart 1: Protocol for management of pregnant patient in roadside trauma.

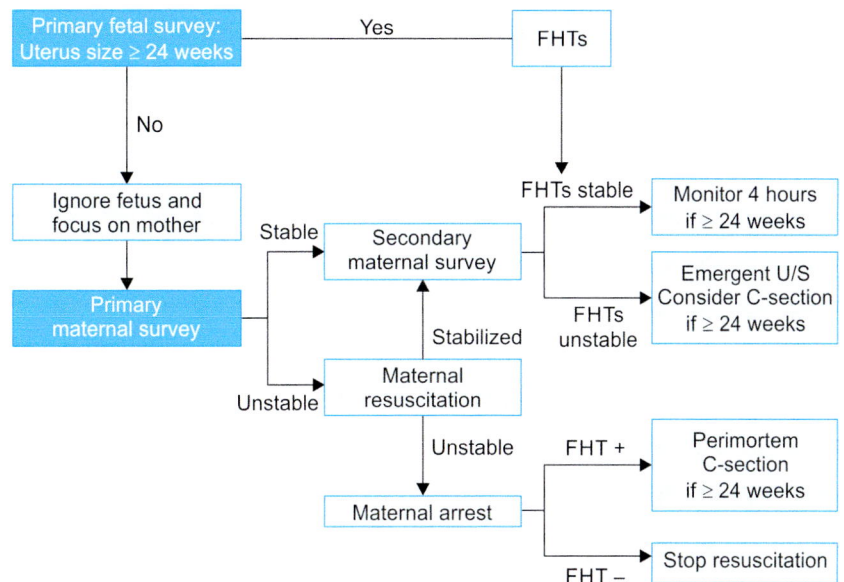

(C-section: cesarean delivery; FTH: fetal heart rate; U/S: ultrasound)

- Patients in the third trimester should be placed in the left lateral position, i.e., on their left side with the right side on top, while being transferred.
- The primary fetal survey should be carried out. If the size of the uterus shows <24 weeks gestation, the fetus should be ignored and the focus should be on the mother.
- If the patient is stable, she should be given first aid and transported to a hospital or nursing home nearby, where fetal monitoring must be done.
- The patient should be shielded with a cloth and then assessed to ascertain the amount of vaginal bleeding. A tense and tender uterus might indicate accidental hemorrhage. The woman must be shifted to a medical center nearby.
- If an obstetric patient has a pelvic injury, the bones must be held in place in the correct position as she is shifted to a hospital. If she is wearing a *dupatta*, it can be wrapped around the lower abdomen.
- A woman who has sustained a trauma in the first trimester of pregnancy is to be treated like any other patient.
- In the case of a woman in the second trimester, the course of action depends on whether or not she is hemodynamically stable. If not, she should be immediately transported to a hospital nearby. If she is hemodynamically stable, the contours of the uterus should be palpated. If normal, she should be transported to a hospital for an ultrasound and fetal and maternal surveillance.
- Rarely, it happens that the patient is already in labor. She should be helped to be in a comfortable position.
- As fetal death is the consequence of maternal death, the main guideline for managing pregnant patients who have sustained trauma is to ensure maternal survival.

SECTION

4

Ward Procedure Skills

Central Venous Line Insertion

Niraj Tyagi

■ INTRODUCTION

A central venous catheter (CVC), mostly called a central line, is an intravascular catheter placed in such a way that the tip lies in one of the venae cavae (close to the center of circulation, i.e., the heart).

■ INDICATIONS

The main indications for the insertion of a CVC are:
- Measurement of central venous pressure
- Infusion of irritant drugs, vasopressors, inotropes, etc.
- Total parenteral nutrition
- Difficult peripheral access
- Hemofiltration
- Hemodialysis
- Insertion of pacing wires or pulmonary artery catheters
- Monitoring of mixed venous or jugular bulb oxygen saturations
- Replacement of circulating volume
- Long-term intravenous treatment (chemotherapy and antibiotics).

■ CATHETER SELECTION

Catheters may be of the following types:
- Single-/multilumen
- Dialysis catheters
- Peripherally inserted central catheters (PICCs)
- Tunneled and implanted ports (for long-term use).

The selection of the catheter should be based upon the reason for the insertion of the CVC and the expected duration for which it is to be used. Catheters with 3–5 lumens are ideal for critically ill patients as they allow for the administration of multiple infusions, however, narrow lumens increase resistance to flow, so such catheters are not suitable for rapid infusion. Larger, shorter catheters, such as an introducer sheath of >7.0 Fr, are more suitable for this purpose. Besides, they also allow for the introduction of devices such as a pulmonary artery catheter.

■ SITE SELECTION

The veins that are commonly accessed are the internal jugular, subclavian, femoral, external jugular, and peripheral/antecubital veins (basilic or cephalic). There is a higher risk of pneumothorax with the subclavian approach, and as the vessels are not accessible to direct compression, this site is least appropriate in patients with severe respiratory disease or bleeding diatheses. Penetrating abdominal trauma or known inferior vena caval disruption would make the femoral approach less desirable.

Internal Jugular Vein

The internal jugular vein (IJV) is the most frequently chosen site for CVC insertion. It has a lower risk of pneumothorax compared to the subclavian approach. A high approach reduces the risk of pneumothorax, but increases the risk of arterial puncture. For lower approaches, the converse is true. Another advantage of this site is that inadvertent arterial puncture can be controlled easily with manual compression. Cannulation can be difficult in patients with very short necks and those who are morbidly obese as landmarks are often obscured.

The IJV descends down the neck in the carotid sheath, with the carotid artery and the vagus nerve. Choosing the right IJV is better because it tends to be larger and straighter than the left. Besides, this avoids the possibility of thoracic duct injury.

Positioning: Make the patient lie supine, with the arms by the sides (if possible, with the head tilting down, to distend the veins, and reduce the risk of air embolism). You may extend the patient's neck by putting a small towel under the shoulders. Turn the head slightly away from the side of cannulation for better access.

Technique: For all approaches, first palpate the carotid artery and ensure that the entry point is lateral to this. Central approach is identify the mastoid process and the sternal head of the sternocleidomastoid (SCM) muscle. The entry level should be the midpoint of the line joining these two landmarks. Insert the needle at 30–40° to the skin, aiming toward the ipsilateral nipple (blood should be obtained within 2.5 cm).

Lateral/posterior approach: The entry point should be roughly 2–3 finger breadths above the clavicle, along the posterior border of the SCM. Direct the needle toward the jugular notch (blood should be aspirated within 5 cm).

Anterior approach: Identify the carotid and the midpoint of the medial SCM border. Aim toward the ipsilateral nipple (blood should be aspirated within 3 cm).

Subclavian Vein

The subclavian vein (SCV) is the continuation of the axillary vein and originates at the lateral border of the first rib. It lies anterior and parallel to the subclavian artery throughout its course. Behind the artery lies the cervical pleura. The SCV has a caliber of 1–2 cm in adults and is thought to be held open by the surrounding tissues even in severe circulatory collapse. It is often preferred for long-term central access as it is generally more comfortable for patients. However,

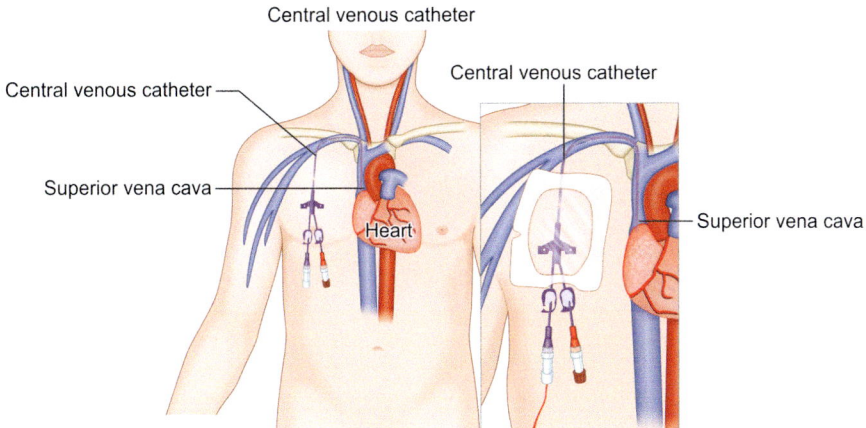

Fig. 1: Central venous line insertion in subclavian vein.

it is best avoided in patients with abnormal clotting or bleeding diatheses as the vessels are inaccessible to direct pressure in case of inadvertent arterial puncture. Pneumothorax is one of the most common major complications associated with this site, with an overall incidence of 1–2%.

Positioning: The patient should be positioned as for the internal jugular approach, with the head tilted down to fill the veins and reduce the risk of air embolism.

Technique: The right SVC is usually preferred as this avoids damage to the thoracic duct. The infraclavicular approach is most commonly used. Insert the needle slightly below the lower border of the middle and medial thirds of the clavicle **(Fig. 1)**. Keep it in the horizontal plane, advancing medially and below the clavicle and aiming for the sternal notch. It should not pass beyond the sternal head of the clavicle.

Femoral Vein

The femoral vein (FV) may be cannulated with the lowest risk of serious short-term complications. This route is useful in urgent situations when the patient is coagulopathic and is perhaps the safest central vein in children in whom peripheral access has failed. However, there is an increased risk of thromboembolic complications, which is why femoral catheters should ideally be removed within 48–72 hours of insertion. The FV starts at the saphenous opening in the thigh and runs alongside the femoral artery to the inguinal ligament, where it becomes the external iliac vein.

Positioning: The patient should be supine with the thigh abducted and externally rotated.

Technique: Palpate the femoral artery 2 cm below the inguinal ligament and insert the needle 1 cm medial while aiming cephalad and slightly medially at an angle of 20–30° to the skin. In adults, the vein is usually 2–4 cm below the skin. In children, it is more superficial so the angle should be 10–15°.

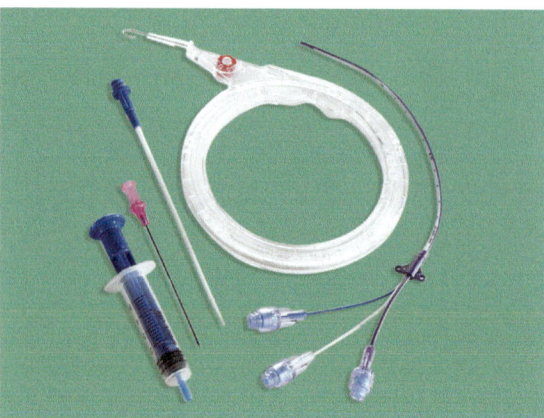

Fig. 2: Equipment necessary for central venous catheter (CVC) insertion.

■ PRINCIPLES OF INSERTION

The basic preparation and equipment required is the same regardless of the site or technique chosen **(Fig. 2)**. Strict asepsis must be maintained at the time of insertion. In nonanesthetized patients, local anesthetic should be used. Chlorhexidine and alcohol solution should be painted over the entirety of the exposed cutaneous surface. Surface anatomical landmarks are essential guides to the relevant deep anatomical structures, so they must remain clearly exposed after preparation and draping.

General Technique

The most common method of insertion is the catheter-over-guidewire (Seldinger) technique.

- The vein is punctured with a small-gauge needle (18 or 20 G) attached to an empty syringe and blood is aspirated. If the blood appears bright red or to be at a high pressure or pulsatile, the possibility of an arterial puncture must be considered.
- The J-tip (to reduce risk of damage to the vessel wall) of the guidewire is passed down the lumen of the needle into the vein and the needle is removed. The guidewire should advance and withdraw easily at all times.
- A dilator is then passed over the guidewire and a small cut made in the skin to allow the dilator to advance a short distance into the vein (further passage along the vein may cause damage to the vessel or distal structures).
- The dilator is then withdrawn and the catheter is threaded on to the guidewire until the end of the guidewire protrudes from the proximal end of the catheter. The end of the guidewire is held while the catheter is advanced to the desired length. Care should be taken not to advance the guidewire with the catheter as this may precipitate arrhythmias and the inadvertent loss of the guidewire intravascularly.
- Finally, the guidewire is removed and the lumens are aspirated and flushed with saline to check for free flow.
- The catheter is secured in place with sutures and a sterile nonocclusive dressing. Antibiotic ointments should not be applied, as they increase the chance of colonization by fungi,

promote the development of antibiotic-resistant bacteria and do not reduce the risk of catheter-related bloodstream infections.

- Ideally, the tip of the catheter should lie at the junction of the superior vena cava and the right atrium. In the case of catheters entering the chest, a chest radiograph should be taken to confirm the position of the tip of the catheter and to rule out complications such as pneumothorax.

■ COMPLICATIONS

Complications can occur in up to 10% of CVCs. The training and experience of the operator are important factors in reducing the rate of complications and experienced help should be sought after repeated attempts. The frequency of mechanical complications is six times greater than after a single attempt.

Pneumothorax (highest for SCV), failure to locate vein, accidental arterial puncture, hemothorax, hematoma, arrhythmias during and postinsertion, thoracic duct injury, and air embolus are some common complications.

■ ULTRASOUND GUIDANCE

Ultrasound imaging should ideally be used to plan and guide all central line insertions to reduce the rate of complications. Real-time sonography provides a means to aim the cannulating needle directly toward the internal jugular, axillary, and femoral veins while avoiding puncture of the accompanying arteries. Given the superficial location of the central veins at the sites of venipuncture, a probe of 7.5 MHz creates optimal images.

■ CONCLUSION

Central venous cannulation has revolutionized patient care for many reasons. While the use of ultrasound localization adds a dimension of orientation, the surface landmarks are still an instrumental component of safe central venous cannulation. Choosing the right site and the right type of catheter along with infection control practices can help minimize complication rates.

Nasogastric Tube and Insertion Technique

Niraj Tyagi, Ashish Dey

■ INTRODUCTION

A nasogastric (NG) tube is a long polyurethane or silicone tube that is passed through the nasal passages, via the esophagus, into the stomach. It may be inserted for prophylactic or therapeutic reasons. It is important to know the correct insertion technique and how to verify the correct positioning.

■ INDICATIONS

The following are the main indications for the insertion of a nasogastric tube:
- To empty the upper gastrointestinal tract in cases of bowel obstruction or decreased motility
- To allow for drainage and/or lavage in drug overdosage or poisoning
- For the assessment of gastrointestinal bleeding in trauma settings or otherwise
- For feeding.

Nasogastric tubes decompress the stomach by releasing air and liquid contents. This is important in the case of patients with ileus, and intestinal and gastric outlet obstruction. These conditions can cause vomiting, which puts patients at risk of aspirating the contents of their stomach contents, leading to potentially lethal pneumonitis.

Nasogastric tubes are useful for feeding patients who have dysphagia, for example after experiencing a stroke, and also for those who have undergone a tracheostomy. Care should be taken in cases where there may be:
- Ear, nose, and throat trauma or infections
- Possible strictures of the esophagus
- Esophageal varices
- Anatomical abnormalities (esophageal diverticula)
- Risk of aspiration
- Severe coagulopathy.

■ SIZES

Nasogastric tubes come in various sizes (8, 10, 12, 14, 16, and 18 Fr). The tube has markings and a radio-opaque marker at the tip so that its position may be checked with the help of X-ray imaging. Stiff tubes are easier to insert, and placing them in a refrigerator or filling them with saline helps to stiffen them further. Some fine-bore tubes come with a guidewire to aid placement.

◼ INSERTION TECHNIQUE

You must explain the details of the insertion procedure to the patient in a reassuring manner before taking his/her verbal consent. Ensure that the trolley prepared for the procedure contains gloves, local anesthetic jelly, or spray, a 60-mL syringe, kidney tray, sticky tape, and a bag to collect secretions. Ideally, the patient should sit up without any head tilt (chin up). Choose a tube of appropriate size and lubricate the tip by smearing aqua gel or a local anesthetic gel (preferably 2% lignocaine). Measure the tubing from the bridge of the nose to the earlobe, and then to the point halfway between the end of the sternum and the navel. Choose the wider nostril and slide the tube down along the floor of the nasal cavity. Patients often gag when the tube reaches the pharynx. Asking them to swallow their saliva or a small amount of water may help to direct the tube into the esophagus. Once the tube is in the esophagus, it may be easy to push it down into the stomach. Do not force the tube. Rotating the head to the contralateral side (of the entrance of the tube) blunts the ipsilateral pyriform sinus, while sniffing position thrusts arytenoid cartilage away from esophageal entrance. If you meet with resistance, rotate the tube slowly with downward advancement toward the ear that is closer.

Withdraw the tube immediately if changes occur in the patient's respiratory status, if the tube coils in the mouth, or if the patient begins to cough. Else, advance the tube until the mark is reached. After verifying the intragastric position of the tube, fix it to the nose and forehead using adhesive tapes. Decompress the stomach by aspirating its contents into a 60-mL syringe attached to the tube.

The use of visualization-aided modalities has been advocated to facilitate NG tube insertion, particularly in intubated and anesthetized patients. The use of GlideScope™ visualization and Macintosh laryngoscope with the assistance of Magill forceps (also is the conventional rescue technique if blind insertion fails) are two options. Failure of bedside NG tube placement is an indication for the use of fluoroscopy or endoscopy.

Verifying Intragastric Position

The intragastric position of the tube must be confirmed after its insertion. Two ways of confirming the tube's position are currently recommended—taking an X-ray and performing a pH test.

Chest X-ray

It is best practice to use X-ray imaging to check the tube's location. This is especially required in the case of patients who have swallowing problems, confused patients, and those in the ICU. The X-ray image should show the chest and the upper half of the abdomen. The tip of the tube, seen as a white radio-opaque line, should be below the diaphragm, on the left side.

pH Test

The NG tube is aspirated and the contents are checked using a pH paper, not a litmus paper. It is safe to feed patients if the pH is 5.5 or below. This advice does not apply in the case of neonates (preterm to 28 days). Proton pump inhibitors or H2 receptor antagonists may alter the pH. Similarly, the intake of milk may neutralize the acid.

Syringe Test

It is also known as the whoosh test, this has been shown to be an unreliable method of checking the placement of the tube and thus, it must not be used.

The intragastric position of the tube should be confirmed:

- Immediately after placement
- Before each feed
- Following vomiting/coughing and when the oxygen saturation decreases
- If the tube is accidentally dislodged or the patient complains of discomfort.

■ COMPLICATIONS

Blind insertion, the most common technique, may result in malposition mucosal trauma if associated with coagulopathy may result in epistaxis following EG tube placement. Nasogastric tubes are often poorly tolerated by conscious patients, since they not only elicit a foreign body sensation in the pharynx, but may also cause reflux esophagitis and pressure ulcers, and have a tendency to dislocate. Infectious complications most frequently seen are aspiration pneumonia.

■ CONCLUSION

Nasogastric tubes are very useful tools in varied clinical situations, provided that the correct insertion technique is used and proper postinsertion care is taken. They are rarely associated with complications and are equally effective as nasojejunal tubes across patient subgroups.

Abdominal Paracentesis and Thoracocentesis

PK Agarwal

■ ABDOMINAL PARACENTESIS

Abdominal paracentesis is a procedure in which fluid from the peritoneal cavity is removed by inserting a needle. The fluid in the abdominal cavity is diagnosed clinically as well as by ultrasound of the abdomen. Diagnostic procedure is done to remove small quantity of ascitic fluid for testing. Therapeutic paracentesis is done to remove large quantity of ascitic fluid (5 L or more). Diagnostic paracentesis is done for evaluation of new onset ascites, preexisting ascites, and ascites with fever, abdominal tenderness, peripheral leukocytosis, and deterioration of hepatic/renal functions or acidosis. Therapeutic or large volume paracentesis is done in tense ascites to reduce intra-abdominal pressure and relieve dyspnea and abdominal distention.

Among the relative contraindications to paracentesis are disseminated intravascular coagulation, primary fibrinolysis and bowel distention and ileus. Ultrasound may be used to avoid intra-abdominal visceral injury. Elevated international normalized ratio (INR) and thrombocytopenia are not contraindication for abdominal paracentesis but fresh frozen plasma or platelets are required in increasing risk of bleeding such as disseminated intravascular coagulation (DIC) or primary fibrinolysis.

For diagnostic paracentesis 1 or 1.5 inch 22-gauze metal needle for average built person and 3.5 inch 22-gauze needle can be used. For therapeutic paracentesis 15- or 16-gauze needle is used. Plastic sheathed needle should be avoided as part of the sheath may be broken into abdominal wall or abdomen during insertion using Z-track technique. After taking informed consent, patient lies in supine position either flat or slightly elevated head end. The common sites for abdominal paracentesis are both flanks and infraumbilical areas in an U-shaped area avoiding superficial veins and surgical scar **(Fig. 1)**. Left lower quadrant of the abdomen is prepared. The needle is attached to 20 mL syringe and advanced through the abdominal wall till it pierces the peritoneum and fluid starts draining into the syringe or may be connected to the gravity assisted system of tubing. After site preparation local anesthetic is injected using z-track technique. Paracentesis needle is then inserted to anesthetized area in z-track technique and fluid is aspirated. For diagnostic test 25 mL of fluid is collected for cell count, cytology, biochemical testing, bacterial culture, and serology. Therapeutic aspiration removal of 5 L or more of ascitic fluid is removed and part of it is sent for testing

Among complications of ascitic tap, ascitic fluid leak, bleeding particularly from vessel in the line of piercing, bowel perforation, and infections are known. Mortality is very low in abdominal paracentesis and if it occurs it is mainly due to bleeding and occasionally due to infection and decompensation of systemic disease.

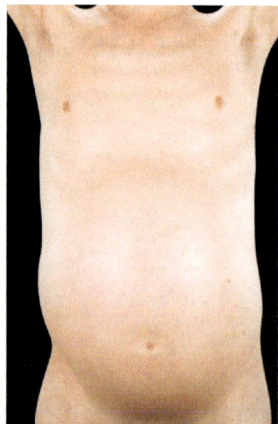

Fig. 1: Sites for abdominal paracentesis.

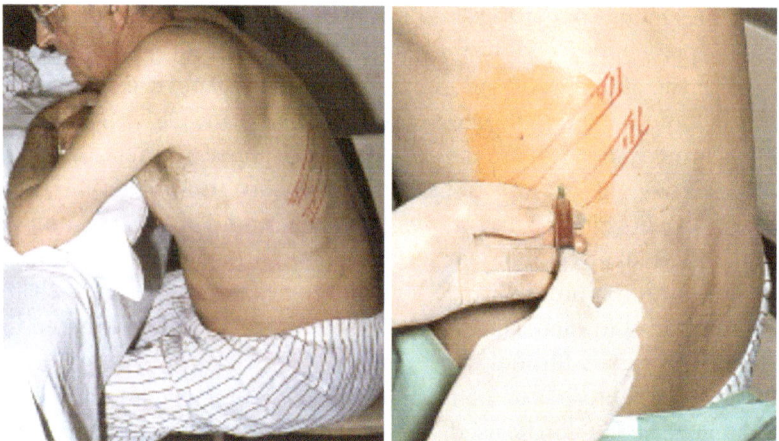

Fig. 2: Site for thoracocentesis.

■ THORACOCENTESIS

Thoracocentesis is percutaneous removal of pleural fluid. Presence of effusion is ascertained clinically and by ultrasound. Diagnostic pleural effusion is done to determine the nature of effusion. Therapeutic thoracocentesis is done by one time needle insertion or putting small bore chest tube or catheter for continuous drainage to drain larger amount of pleural effusion. It is done for symptomatic relief or in management of complicated pleural effusion.

Contraindication for pleural tapping or thoracocentesis is presence of insignificant pleural fluid, bleeding diathesis, skin infection, and inflammation. Mechanical ventilation or positive end-expiratory pressure (PEEP) is not a contraindication to thoracocentesis.

After taking informed consent for thoracocentesis from patient and/or attendants of the patient, the patient is positioned in upright sitting position with the arms resting on the surface **(Fig. 2)**. Thoracocentesis is done under ultrasound guidance at the bed site or procedure room. CT guidance is required in failed ultrasound-guided tap or in small, loculated pleural effusion.

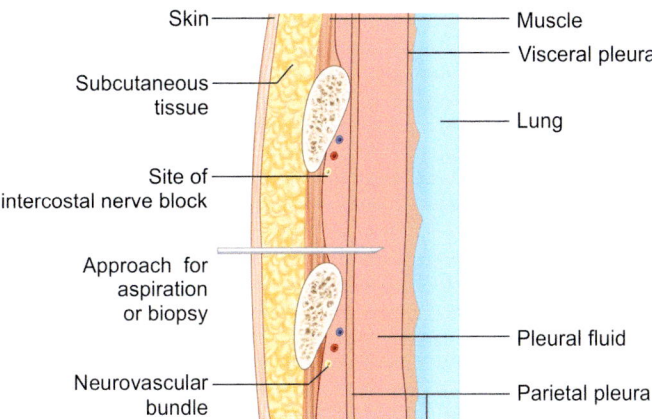

Skin — Muscle
Visceral pleura
Subcutaneous tissue
Lung
Site of intercostal nerve block
Approach for aspiration or biopsy
Pleural fluid
Neurovascular bundle
Parietal pleura

Fig. 3: Needle insertion in thoracocentesis.

The thoracocentesis site guided by ultrasound is usually lower posterior intercostal space in upright position. After identifying puncture site and local sterilization, local anesthesia is injected using 20–22-gauge needle. A 16- or 18-size needle with catheter is used for one time drainage **(Fig. 3)**; however, intercostal drainage kit is used for ICD. Three-way stopcock is used for syringe drainage, but gravity drainage or vacuum bottle drainage for ICD is used. The test performed as pleural fluid includes cell count, cytology, biochemical test, Gram stain, and culture. Fluid is also examined for turbidity, color, and coagulation. Once the required amount of pleural fluid is drained, catheter is removed with stopcock and syringe still attached to it while patient holds the breath. Local pressure is put at the site and later occlusive dressing is placed. Among the complications of pleural tapping or thoracocentesis is dry tap, needle/catheter blockage, visceral pleural impingement, pneumothorax, infection, liver or spleen puncture, and bleeding. Following thoracocentesis patient to be examined clinically and if required or check chest X-ray may be done to rule out pneumothorax.

Epistaxis

Devinder Rai

■ INTRODUCTION

Epistaxis or bleeding from the nose can have a myriad causes. The bleeding can be of any intensity. If it is profuse, it has the potential of exsanguinating the patient, with serious consequence. It has to be managed on a case-to-case basis. One of the extremely important procedures that is required to be known is that of nasal packing.

■ ASSESSMENT

Make an assessment the moment the patient arrives.
- If the bleeding has stopped, take a detailed history and conduct a physical examination.
- If there is active bleeding, make an assessment in accordance with the condition while trying to control the bleeding.

Control of Bleeding

The instant 9 minutes compress:
- Seat the patient on a chair with the head tilted forward and a bowl under the chin. The patient should not lie down because blood may then trickle into the throat.
- Ask the patient to breathe through the mouth
- Compress the anterior cartilaginous part of the nose (just below the nasal bones) between the forefinger and the thumb. This compresses the Little's area (Kiesselbach's plexus) on the septum.
- Continue compressing with an even pressure for 9 minutes by the clock, as this is the usual bleeding/clotting time for most people. Do not release the pressure to check if the bleeding has stopped because if it recurs, you will have to start the timing all over again.
- The application of a cold compress may help, though this is debatable.

If not successful:
This method is often referred to as Trotter's method. However, in Trotter's method, bleeding was allowed to continue and the blood pressure of the patient to drop until the bleeding stopped. This at times led to severe exsanguination and consequent hypovolemic shock.

■ NASAL PACKING

If the bleeding does not stop in 9 minutes, use nasal packing. You will require the following:
- Tilley's nasal packing forceps

- Nasal speculum
- Tongue depressor
- 1/0 silk on needle
- Suction apparatus with catheters or/and suction tips/cannulas.

Material

- Sterile gauze cut to size and rolled
- Two pieces of sterile ribbon gauze (width: 1 cm and length: 1 m) impregnated with a paraffin-based antibiotic cream/petroleum jelly/mixture of Betadine solution and paraffin
- Sofra-Tulle gauze
- Plain gauze
- 4% topical lignocaine.

Importance of Suturing the Packs

The end of every piece is sutured by a 1/0 silk, which is kept long (about 20 cm). After the nasal packs are in the nostrils, tie the individual sutures to each other and tape the combined thread assembly to the side of the nostril with an adhesive hypoallergenic tape. This prevents the gauze pieces from sliding into the throat and obstructing the larynx, which could lead to fatal respiratory obstruction.

Anterior Nasal Packing Technique

- The patient should be supine with the head raised at 30°.
- Spray the nostrils with 4% lignocaine
- Wear gloves and mask
- Examine the nose with a nasal speculum and headlight
- Suck out the blood and/or blood clots if feasible, depending on the bleeding intensity
- Ascertain the site of bleeding, if feasible
- Hold the medicated ribbon gauze approximately 10–20 cm from the end with the nasal packing forceps
- Insert the ribbon gauze in the two layers thus formed, hugging the floor of the nostril right up to the posterior nares
- Take out the nasal forceps, pressing the ribbon gauze sequentially as you withdraw
- Then hold the ribbon gauze about 5–15 cm outside the nose and insert it over the first two layers, without dislodging them, going all the way back as before
- Pack the nostril in layers, shortening the ribbon gauze each time
- While packing, remember that the vault of the nostril is shaped like a dome. If you do not pack adequately, you may miss the anterior/posterior ethmoidal artery as it traverses high up.
- In cases of nasal or maxillofacial trauma, be gentle as the base of the skull may be fractured and you may introduce the nasal pack into the cranium if you use force.
- Repeat the procedure on the other nostril even if it is not bleeding, to provide counter pressure to the pack on the bleeding side.

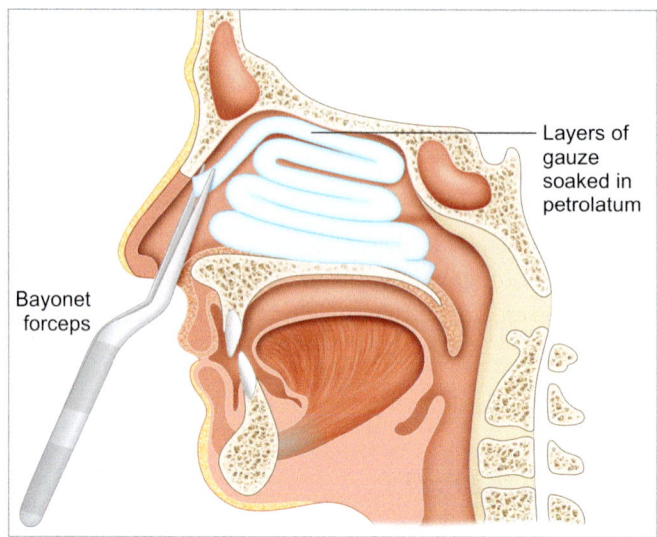

Fig. 1: Anterior nasal packing for epistaxis.

- Place a gauze pack over the nose, covering the anterior nares. Secure it with two hypoallergenic adhesive tapes, one under the anterior nares and one across the dorsum of the nose in its caudal aspect. Make it tight to provide extra pressure **(Fig. 1)**.
- Check the throat for bleeding and any piece of gauze dropping into the oropharynx and review after about 15 minutes.

In an Emergency

Sometimes, you may need to tackle nasal bleeding outside the OPD/hospital. In that case, look around you to find something suitable. You may, for example, use a clean handkerchief or cotton wool as the nasal packing material, and eyebrow tweezers instead of nasal forceps.

Posterior Nasal Packing

Fashioning the Nasal Pack

Roll and wrap a piece of gauze around itself tightly. The size should be approximately that of the first digit of the patient's thumb. Secure it with 1/0 silk suturing—let the needle go through the pack, pass the thread around the pack and knot it. Keep the two threads long (about 30 cm). Pass another suture through the pack and knot it, but only one thread is retained and kept long (30 cm). Impregnate the pack with liquid paraffin and Betadine or a petroleum-based antibiotic ointment.

Technique

- Ask the patient to sit up to reduce the chances of choking. However, the patient could be supine if that is not possible.
- Wear a mask, protective glasses or visor and gown

- Spray the nostrils with 4% lignocaine
- Pass a flexible nasal catheter through each of the nostrils and bring them out through the mouth
- Tie the catheters to the long silk threads sutured to the pack, and manipulate the pack into the nasopharynx
- There is a risk of the pack getting stuck at the palatal level. If this happens, pull the catheters gently and swing the pack into the nasopharynx digitally.
- The patient experiences discomfort at this juncture and may cough or spit out blood. Protect your eyes, face, and body from getting splashed with blood by wearing protective glasses, mask, and gown.
- Secure the third thread on the cheek with an adhesive. The nasopharyngeal pack is removed by pulling this thread, usually after 48–72 hours.

ADDITIONAL/ANCILLARY TREATMENT

Foley's catheter may be used instead of the posterior nasal gauze pack.

- Lubricate a Foley's catheter with an appropriate xylocaine jelly and insert it into the bleeding nostril.
- Inflate it with about 10–20 mL air with the help of a syringe. Some physicians prefer to inflate it with water, but if it bursts inside the nasopharynx, it may result in aspiration.
- Pull the catheter to exert traction. It should abut the posterior nares snugly.
- Knot and support the catheter in such a way that it does not come in contact with the columellar and alar tissue to prevent pressure necrosis.
- Tape the catheter on the cheek or forehead with the help of adhesive hypoallergenic plaster.
- Before removing the catheter, deflate the bulb and watch for 6–24 hours. This way, the catheter can be conveniently inflated if there is any bleeding.
- Remove the anterior nasal packing if there is no bleeding subsequently. In cases of emergency, modifications of the technique may be used with readily available materials as shown in **Figure 2**.

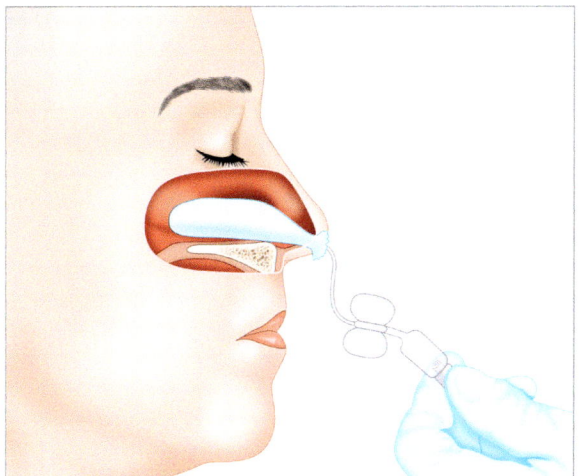

Fig. 2: Nasal packing for severe nosebleeds.

Absorbent Expandable Nasal Tampon

You may use a sterile nasal tampon, preferably with a suture attached to it. It expands when saline or an antibiotic eye drop is introduced. Though such tampons are expensive and may not exert the requisite pressure, they are easier to place.

- Select one which has an attached silk thread and smear it with a paraffin- or petroleum jelly-based ointment.
- Do not irrigate it at this time
- Hold it with nasal packing forceps or with your thumb and forefinger
- Use a nasal speculum or tilt the tip of the nose upward
- Slide the tampon along the floor of the nose
- Sometimes, you may require another tampon. Direct the second tampon upward, toward the vault of the nose.
- Irrigate the tampon with normal saline or an antibiotic eye drop
- Repeat the procedure on the other side.
- If you suspect a posterior nasal bleed, push the first tampon into the nasopharynx through the posterior nares
- You may require two or even three tampons for each side.
- Remember to tie the threads to each other and then secure the bunch over the dorsum of the nose with a hypoallergenic adhesive tape
- Use a gauze to bolster the pressure as mentioned earlier.

◼ WHEN TO REFER

You must refer the patient for specialized care:

- If the bleeding is intractable
- In case of recurrent bleeding
- If the patient is a boy in the age group of 5–18 years as the cause may be an angiofibroma.
- If you suspect tumor
- If the patient is suffering from cardiac or respiratory conditions.
- In case of nasal trauma.

38 Fine-needle Aspiration Cytology

Sunita Bhalla

■ HISTORY OF ASPIRATION BIOPSY

The first report on the use of "needle puncture" can be found in the Kitab al-Tasrif (The Method of Medicine), the most influential book of Arab medieval medicine. The author, Albucasis or Abu al-Qasim Khalaf ibn al-Abbas (936–1013), described fine-needle aspiration (FNA) of the thyroid gland, employing instruments resembling the modern aspiration needle. In 1847, Kun described the use of a needle as a "new instrument for the diagnosis of tumors". Dudgeon and Patrick (1927) in the UK and Martin and Ellis (1930) at New York's Memorial Hospital for Cancer and Allied Diseases are generally credited with the first description of the sampling of tumors by means of a narrow-gauge needle.

In the 1950s and 1960s, there was increasing interest in the FNA technique in northern Europe and Scandinavia. Hematopathologists such as Soderstrom and Franzen in Sweden and Lopes Cardozo in Holland were prominent among those who furthered the field. They introduced the use of higher gauge needles (22-gauge or higher) for performing aspiration, as opposed to the standard 18-gauge needle that had been used previously in the USA. In addition, they defined precise diagnostic criteria to be applied to aspiration biopsies, increasing the sensitivity and specificity of the procedure. The Swedish experience with FNA of tumor lesions of the breast, salivary gland and thyroid in the 1960s and 1970s served as a model for the development of FNA clinics throughout the world. Since the 1970s, improvements in imaging, including computed tomography scan and ultrasound, in combination with the development of new specialties such as interventional radiology have led to an increase in the use of FNA among clinicians and radiologists.

■ EQUIPMENT (FIG. 1)

Needles

Standard disposable needles of 27–22 gauge (0.4–0.7 mm) and 30–50 mm length are suitable for superficial and palpable lesions. A 27-gauge needle is usually used when aspirating vascular organs, such as the thyroid, and small cutaneous lesions. Twenty-two-gauge, 90-mm-long disposable lumbar puncture needles with a trocar, or 22-gauge, 150- or 250-mm-long Chiba needles are used for deep biopsies. They are sufficiently rigid and the trocar prevents contamination during the passage of the needle through the surrounding tissues.

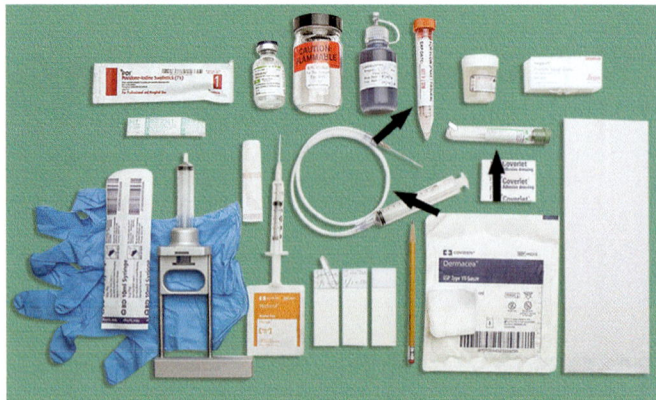

Fig. 1: Materials for fine-needle aspiration cytology (FNAC).

Syringes and Syringe Holder

Standard disposable plastic syringes mounted in a syringe holder/pistol grip are suitable for conventional aspiration biopsy.

Containers and Slides

Small sterile containers which have tight lids and contain physiological saline or a transport medium, such as Hank's balanced salt solution, should be at hand if a cell suspension or a cell block is needed. The glass slides must be clean, dry and free of grease. Slides with frosted ends are convenient for immediate labeling.

Fixatives and Stains

Smears are air-dried or wet-fixed. For routine wet fixation, you can use either 70–90% ethanol or a commercial spray fixative.

Other

Among the other things that should be available on the biopsy tray, tool box, or trolley are skin disinfectant (preinjection swabs), sterile dressings, a local anesthetic, tongue depressors, a small electric torch, and sterile scalpel blades (to scrape smears from skin or mucous membranes). Latex gloves and face masks may be required for safety reasons.

■ PREPARATION OF PATIENT

Patients should be asked for their consent and the procedure should be clearly explained to them to reassure them and gain their cooperation. A formal written consent may be required, at least for deep biopsies. Using prepacked swabs to disinfect the area is adequate for biopsies of superficial lesions. The preparations for transpleural, transperitoneal, and bone biopsies are similar to those recommended for minor surgical procedures (surgical skin disinfectant, fenestrated sterile cloth, and sterile gloves).

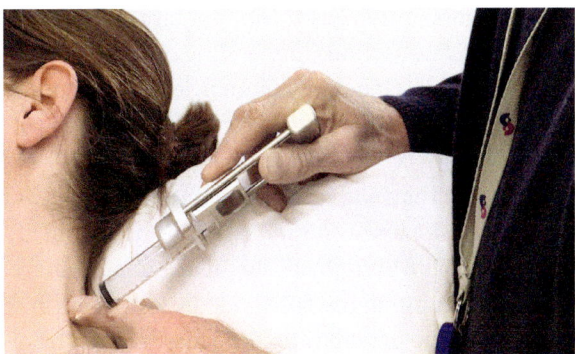

Fig. 2: Technique of fine-needle aspiration cytology.

■ PROCEDURE (FIG. 2)

It is imperative to examine the patient and palpate the lesion. This is the time to plan the procedure, locate the lesion, and estimate the depth of the lesion. Decide on the best angle and entry point to access the lesion while minimizing the amount of soft tissue the needle will traverse before entering the lesion. Most often, the needle should enter perpendicular to the skin surface and lesion.

Insertion of Needle

You should use universal infection precautions. The first step in performing an FNA procedure is to palpate and stabilize the lesion with one hand, typically with two fingers, or push the lesion into a fixed position. Prepare the surface of the skin at the site of needle puncture with an alcohol sponge, place the needle against the skin at a predetermined angle, and then insert it through the skin and into the subcutaneous tissue in a swift smooth motion.

Fine-needle Biopsy with Aspiration

Once you have positioned the needle within the target tissue, pull the plunger to apply negative pressure. Along with persistent application of negative pressure, move the needle back and forth inside the target to increase the yield. You must release the negative pressure before withdrawing the needle. If negative pressure is maintained, it may cause contamination along the track by the material aspirated when the needle is being withdrawn while the needle remains in the target tissue. Next, detach the needle and draw air into the syringe. Finally, blow the sample onto the microscopy slide. The negative pressure does not tear cells from the tissue, but merely holds the tissue against the sharp cutting edge of the needle, which scrapes or cuts softer tissue components along the track as it advances through the tissue.

Fine-needle Sampling without Aspiration

Fine-needle biopsy (FNB) without aspiration was introduced by Zajdela in 1987. This technique is based on the observation that the capillary pressure in a fine needle is sufficient to keep the detached cells inside its lumen. In this procedure, you have to hold a 23–27-gauge standard needle directly with your fingers and insert it into the target tissue. Next, move it back and forth in several directions for a few seconds, depending on the cellularity and the vascularity of the tissue, and then withdraw it. Generally, there is less admixture with blood than in the case of aspiration. The technique is particularly well suited for biopsy of the thyroid and other vascular tissues.

The cell yield may be smaller than with aspiration, but not significantly so.

When using FNA for deep lesions, you should use anesthesia. Mostly, you will need to use an 18-gauge guide needle. Place it within the lesion, using imaging to verify its position. Then insert a 21- or 22-gauge needle through the guide needle and confirm the position within the lesion. Obtain the sample while the patient is holding his/her breath to reduce trauma and, in the case of the lungs, to reduce the risk of pneumothorax. In cases of endoscopic US-FNA, use endoscopic ultrasound to target the lesion and position the endoscope at the site of the lesion. To identify the vascular anatomy and prevent the insertion of the needle into vessels within the projected needle path, use color Doppler imaging. Next, pass the needle-catheter assembly through the biopsy channel of the echoendoscope. Advance the needle under endoscopic ultrasound guidance to the middle of the lesion with a quick, firm thrust of the handle. When the needle has been clearly placed in the target lesion, push the stylet to the tip of the needle and then withdraw it completely. Attach a syringe to the head of the needle device and oscillate the needle back and forth within the lesion approximately 10–20 times with suction. Release the suction, withdraw the needle into the catheter, and remove the whole system from the echoendoscope.

Direct Smearing

The quality of the smear depends to a great extent on whether the smear is thin and evenly spread, ideally as a monolayer of cells. The optimal sample, obtainable from cell-rich tissues, has a creamy consistency due to high cellularity and little or no blood or fluid ("dry" sample). It is best if you smear a "dry" sample with the flat of a second slide, exerting light pressure as you move it along the specimen slide. Adjust the pressure carefully to achieve a thin and even spread, without causing disruption of tissue fragments with loss of microarchitecture, or smudging artifacts. Optimal smearing is a fine balance between too thick and too thin.

Indirect Smearing

Thin watery samples are processed by centrifugation in a cytocentrifuge. Some laboratories prefer to rinse needles and syringes routinely with saline or a fixative, which is then centrifuged or filtered onto slides.

◼ TISSUE FRAGMENTS AND CELL BLOCKS

Sometimes, you obtain a thin core or fragments of tissue with a standard 22-gauge needle. Tissue fragments are fixed in 5–10% buffered isotonic formalin and processed as for routine histology. Some laboratories recommend the routine preparation of cell blocks for paraffin embedding of FNB samples. Cell blocks may give you a better idea of tissue architecture and allow for multiple sections for panels of immune markers with controls.

■ FIXATION AND STAINING

Two fundamentally different methods of fixation and staining are used in fine-needle aspiration cytology (FNAC). One is air-drying followed by a Romanowsky-type and alcohol-fixation followed by Papanicolaou (Pap). The other is hematoxylin and eosin (H&E) staining. Both methods have their advantages and deficiencies. Air-drying causes the cell, both cytoplasm and nucleus, to flatten on the slide as an egg flattens in the frying pan. It, therefore, appears larger than an ethanol-fixed cell, which maintains its three-dimensional shape.

■ SPECIAL STAINS

The special stains commonly used in histopathology are also used for cytological smears, without major modifications. Some examples are PAS/diastase or Alcian blue for mucins, Prussian blue for iron, Masson-Fontana for melanin, Grimelius for argyrophilic granules, and Congo red for amyloid.

■ IMMUNOCYTOCHEMISTRY

Probably the most important recent development in diagnostic cytology is the increasing commercial availability of monoclonal antisera to a variety of proteins and other cell products that are more or less specific to different cell lines. The demonstration and identification of such cell products in smears and cell blocks is of immense value as it offers a means of objectively recognizing the line of differentiation shown by the cells. Immunostaining may allow you to confidently make a specific diagnosis even on the basis of relatively scanty material. Immune markers are extremely useful for differentiating between anaplastic carcinoma, neuroendocrine tumors, malignant lymphoma, and amelanotic melanoma. They also help in the search for a primary in metastatic malignancies (e.g., differential staining for a number of cytokeratins), and in the histogenetic typing of mesenchymal tumors. Markers for B and T cells, immunoglobulins and light chains are indispensable to the typing of lymphoma. Monoclonal antibodies to certain tumor antigens have been found to be useful in the distinction between malignant and benign epithelial cells.

■ SUGGESTED READING

1. Akhtar SS, Imran-Ul-Huq, Faiz-U-Din M, Reyes LM. Efficacy of fine-needle capillary biopsy in the assessment of patients with superficial lymphadenopathy. Cancer. 1997; 81:277-80.
2. Aspegren K, Biorklund A, Soderstrom N, Akerman M. et al. Fine-needle biopsy in thyroid carcinoma. Lakartidningen. 1976;73: 730-2.
3. Bell DA, Carr CP, Szyfelbein WM. Fine needle aspiration cytology of focal liver lesions. Results obtained with examination of both cytologic and histologic preparations. Acta Cytol. 1986;30:397-402.
4. Berger T, Soderstrom N. Fine-needle aspiration biopsy in diseases of the salivary glands. Acta Pathol Microbiol Scand. 1963; 58:1-9.
5. Boon ME, Lykles C. Imaginative approach to fine needle aspiration cytology. Lancet. 1980;2:1031-2.
6. Campbell F, Herrington CS. Application of cytokeratin 7 and 20 immunohistochemistry to diagnostic pathology. Curr Diagn Pathol. 2001;7:113-22.

7. Davidson DD, Goheen MP. Preparation of fine needle aspiration biopsies for electron microscopy. In: Schmidt WA (Ed). Cytopathology Annual. Baltimore: Williams and Wilkins; 1993. pp. 255-64.

8. de Boer WB, Segal A, Frost FA, Sterrett GF. Can CD34 discriminate between benign and malignant hepatocytic lesions in fine-needle aspirates and thin core biopsies? Cancer. 2000;90:273-8.

9. Diamantis A, Magiorkinis E, Koutselini H. Fine-needle aspiration (FNA) biopsy: Historical aspects. Folia Histochem Cytobiol. 2009;47:191-7.

10. Dudgeon LS, Patrick CV. A new method for the rapid microscopical diagnosis of tumours. Br J Surg. 1927;15:250-61.

11. Franzen S, Zajicek J. Aspiration biopsy in the diagnosis of palpable lesions of the breast. Acta Radiol. 1968;7:214-62.

12. Guidelines of the Papanicolaou Society of Cytopathology for fine-needle aspiration procedure and reporting. The Papanicolaou Society of Cytopathology Task Force on Standards of Practice. Diagn Cytopathol. 1997;17:239-47.

13. Gupta S, Henningsen JA, Wallace MJ, Madoff DC, Morello FA Jr, Ahrar K, et al. Percutaneous biopsy of the head and neck lesions the CT guidance: Various approaches and relevant anatomic and technical considerations. Radiographics. 2007;27:371-90.

14. Haack LA, Meier JS, Gluth J, Selvaggi SM. The other side of the needle: A patient's perspective. Diagn Cytopathol. 2006;34: 303-6.

15. Irisawa A, Hikichi T, Bhutani MS, Ohira H. Basic technique of FNA. Gastrointest Endosc. 2009;69(2 Suppl):S125-9.

16. Kate MS, Kamal MM, Bobhate SK, Kher AV. Evaluation of fine needle capillary sampling in superficial and deep-seated lesions. An analysis of 670 cases. Acta Cytol. 1998;42:679-84.

17. Martin HE, Ellis EB. Biopsy by needle puncture and aspiration. Ann Surg. 1930; 92:169-81.

18. Nathan NA, Narayan E, Smith MM, Horn MJ. Cell block cytology. Improved preparation and its efficacy in diagnostic cytology. Am J Clin Pathol. 2000;114:599-606.

19. Osborn M, Domagala W. Immunocytochemistry. In: Bibbo M (Ed). Comprehensive Cytopathology, 2nd edition. Philadelphia: Saunders; 1997.

20. Polak J, van Noorden S. Introduction to immunocytochemistry. In: Current techniques and problems, 2nd edition. Berlin: Springer-Verlag; 1997.

21. Sachdeva R, Kline TS. Aspiration biopsy cytology and special stains. Acta Cytol. 1981;25:678-83.

22. Sirkin W, Auger M, Donat E, Lipa M. Cytospins—an alternative method for fine-needle aspiration cytology of the breast: A study of 148 cases. Diagn Cytopathol. 1995; 13:266-9.

23. Soderstrom N, Telenius-Berg M, Akerman M. Diagnosis of medullary carcinoma of the thyroid by fine-needle aspiration biopsy. Acta Med Scand. 1975;197:71-6.

24. Soderstrom N. Fine-needle aspiration biopsy. Stockholm: Almqvist and Wiksell; 1966.

25. Suthipintawong C, Leong AS, Vinyuvat S. Immunostaining of cell preparations: A comparative evaluation of common fixatives and protocols. Diagn Cytopathol. 1996; 15:167-74.

26. Thompson P. Thin needle aspiration biopsy. Acta Cytologica. 1982;26: 262-3.

27. Van Hoeven KH, Fitzpatrick BT, Bibbo M. Update of immunocytochemistry in cytopathology. In: Rosen PP, Fechner RE (Eds). Pathology Annual, Vol.30, Part 2. Stanford: Appleton and Lange; 1995.

28. Vilman P, Săftoiu A. Endoscopic ultrasoundguided fine-needle aspiration biopsy: Equipment and technique. J Gastroenterol Hepatol. 2006;21:1646-55.

29. Zajdela A, Zillhardt P, Voillemot N. Cytological diagnosis by fine needle sampling without aspiration. Cancer. 1987;59:1201-5.

Intra-articular Aspiration, Injection, and Soft Tissue Injection

Lalit Duggal

■ INTRODUCTION

Injection procedures are useful adjuncts to treatments for various types of musculoskeletal pain. They are quite safe in the hands of a skilled doctor who knows how to handle a needle to be inserted into a joint. Synovial aspiration is important diagnostically and therapeutically. There are various indications for joint and soft tissue injections in rheumatological conditions. Most of the time, the joint is aspirated before the intra-articular injection is administered to curb any underlying inflammatory process, after ruling out infection.

Although joint and soft tissue aspiration/injection are being performed under ultrasound guidance nowadays, they can easily be performed as a blind procedure by an experienced doctor who is familiar with the anatomical landmarks and techniques of administering injections. The patient should be calm and restful for at least 10 minutes before the procedure. In the case of the lower limb joints, ask the patient to lie down. When the upper limb joints are involved, instruct the patient to sit up with his/her arms resting on a table. All the necessary equipment should be ready before the procedure. This includes gloves, forceps, povidone iodine, alcohol swabs, adequate gauze and cotton, Band-Aid, local anesthetic (lignocaine), culture bottles, culture plates, test tubes, and medicines such as methylprednisolone, triamcinolone, and viscosupplements.

Explain the details of the procedure to the patient and obtain his/her written consent before the procedure. Follow the universally accepted precautions from the first step to the last. You must adhere to the standard guidelines for biowaste management.

■ BASICS OF INTRA-ARTICULAR TECHNIQUES

In the case of anxious patients, administer a 1% or 2% lignocaine injection subcutaneously following proper painting and draping. Clean the surface of the skin with an alcohol swab and apply povidone iodine. For small joints, use a 23–27-gauge needle, while for large joints such as the knee and shoulder, use a 20–21-gauge needle. Many times during the aspiration of fluid, debris gets lodged in the needle tract. This problem can be overcome by slight withdrawal/ rotation of the needle or even reinjection of some fluid. You should not change the needle for aspiration, i.e., administer the injection using the same needle. It is extremely important to have a tight and stable hold over the needle during aspiration and injection.

After the procedure has been completed, remove the needle swiftly and apply light pressure over the area where the needle pierced the skin. Cover the area with a Band-Aid for a few hours. After an intra-articular injection, you should advise the patient to move the joint concerned. This will facilitate the uniform spread of the medicine in the joint. All patients should be advised not to strain for at least 24 hours and to rest the injected joint. You can prescribe the local application of a cold pack 3–4 times a day or the use of NSAIDs as and when required (on an SOS basis) for postinjection pain, prevention, and treatment.

■ INDICATIONS

Diagnostic Purposes

- To evaluate monoarthritis/suspected septic arthritis
- To rule out crystal arthropathy
- To differentiate between primary tuberculosis of a joint, Poncet's arthritis or reactive arthritis
- To diagnose tumors/malignancies, e.g., pigmented villonodular synovitis.

Therapeutic Purposes

- Injection of steroids for osteoarthritis
- Injection of viscosupplementation or platelet-rich plasma for early osteoarthritis
- Injection of steroids for rheumatoid arthritis (RA), spondyloarthritis, and joints affected by gout that are unresponsive to the usual treatments [disease-modifying antirheumatic drugs, biologics, systemic steroids, colchicine, nonsteroidal anti-inflammatory drugs (NSAIDs)]
- Medical synovectomy (synoviorthesis) in RA, osteoarthritis, hemophilia, pigmented villonodular arthropathy, or other chronic inflammatory conditions leading to joint effusion
- Treatment of frozen shoulder
- Treatment of Baker's cysts.

■ CONTRAINDICATIONS

- Local skin infection or generalized skin disorder
- Sepsis/septic shock
- Bleeding diathesis/severe thrombocytopenia
- Immunocompromised state
- Best avoided in patients with joint prostheses.

■ COMPLICATIONS

The complications, which are very rare and never life-threatening, are as follows:
- Vasovagal syncope
- Local bleeding
- Infection, especially with steroid injections
- Steroid arthropathy in patients who have repeatedly taken intra-articular steroid injections
- Transient hyperglycemia (for 2–3 days, especially among diabetics) and deranged hypothalamus–pituitary–adrenal axis (for at least 1–2 weeks)

- Facial flush, rash, allergic reactions, and an extremely rare chance of anaphylactic shock
- Tendon rupture, skin atrophy, fat atrophy, nerve damage, vein, or artery puncture
- Postinjection flare—exacerbation of pain induced by corticosteroid crystals hours after injection that may last for a few days

■ INJECTION TECHNIQUES (FIGS. 1A TO F)

Joint Injections

For the proximal interphalangeal, metacarpophalangeal, and metatarsophalangeal joints, use 10 mg methylprednisolone. It is best to avoid triamcinolone since it can lead to postinjection pigmentation and atrophy. Use the dorsolateral approach, with the finger in a semiflexed position. It is possible to inject several small joints in a single session.

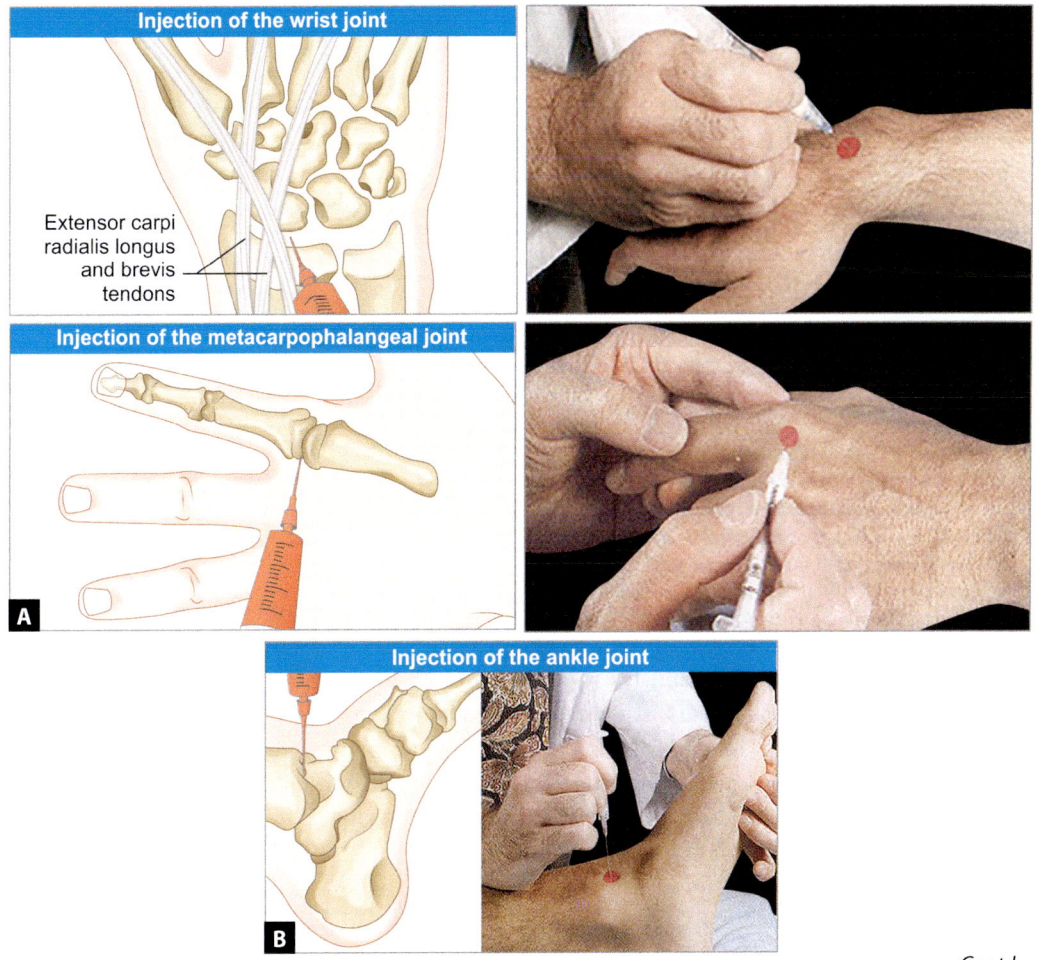

Injection of the wrist joint

Extensor carpi radialis longus and brevis tendons

Injection of the metacarpophalangeal joint

A

Injection of the ankle joint

B

Contd...

Figs. 1A and B

Contd...

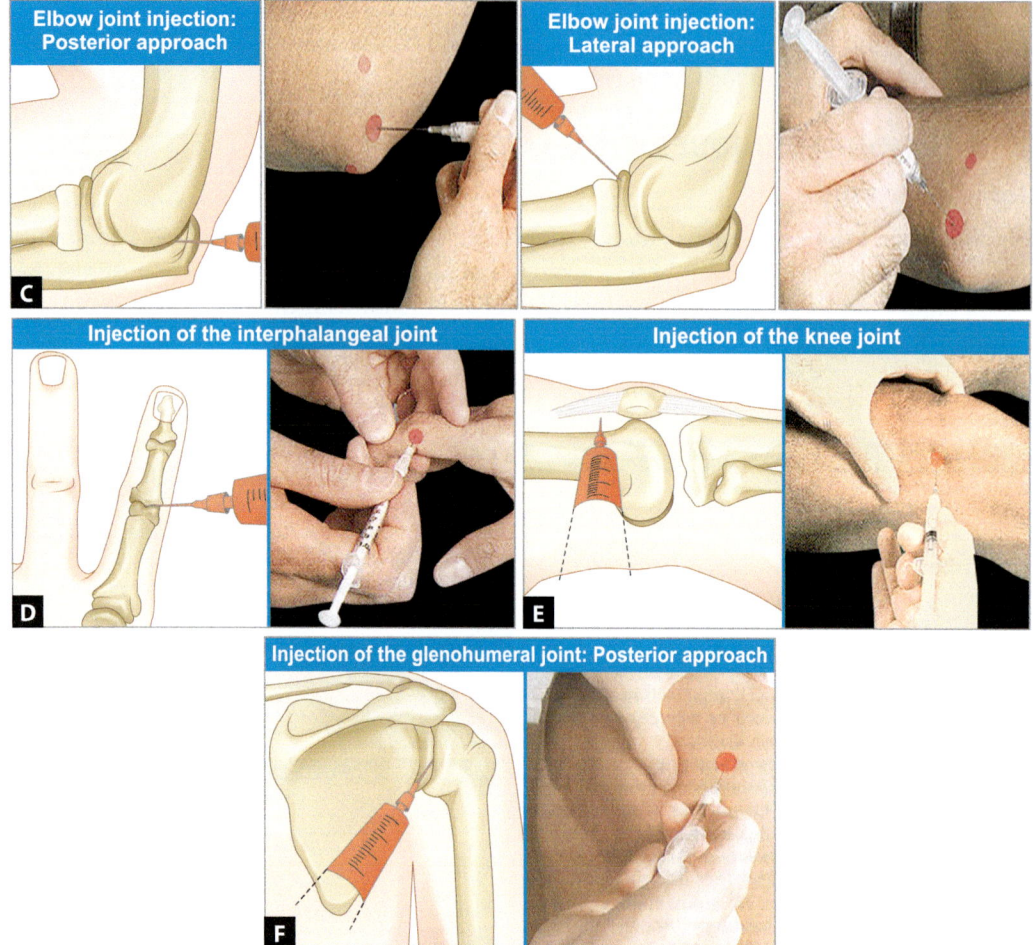

Figs. 1A to F: Injection techniques of various joints.

When dealing with the wrist joint, you must first identify Lister's tubercle and using a dorsal approach, inject 20–40 mg methylprednisolone just distal to Lister's tubercle.

Two approaches can be used for injecting the elbow—lateral and posterior. In both approaches, the elbow is held in flexion at 90°. For a lateral entry, palpate the radial head and insert the needle just proximal to it. When using the posterior approach, palpate the tip of the olecranon and mentally draw an imaginary line that joins the medial and lateral epicondyles. Insert the needle just below the line and just above the tip of the olecranon, and inject 20–40 mg of methylprednisolone/triamcinolone.

For the shoulder, you may use either the posterior or anterior approach, though the former is the preferred one. Ask the patient to be seated and palpate the posterior margin of the acromion. Insert the needle 1 cm below and 1 cm medial to the posterior angle of the acromion, and direct the needle anteromedially. You can also use an anterior approach, with the patient in a sitting position, his/her arms hanging down and the elbow flexed at a 90° angle. Palpate the coracoid process and insert the needle anteroposteriorly, 1 cm distal and 1 cm lateral to the coracoid process. Once the needle hits the bone, joint is passively internally rotated to make the needle's way into the joint.

Injections in the hip joint are usually administered under ultrasound guidance. But if necessary, they can be given blindly, using a 26- or 27-gauge lumbar puncture needle. You have to first mark the greater trochanter, and then the anterior superior iliac spine (ASIS). Next, make a horizontal line passing through the ASIS and a vertical one passing through the greater trochanter. These lines form two arms of a triangle. Draw a third line joining both landmarks. Insert the needle at the medial one-third of the third line, making sure that the direction of the needle is toward the meeting point of the first two lines. You may inject 40–60 mg methylprednisolone.

For knee joints, the patient should be in a supine position. Insert the needle under the surface of the patella, midway between its upper and lower poles. You can approach from the lateral or medial aspects of the knee joint. After aspirating the fluid, you may inject 40–80 mg methylprednisolone.

In the case of the ankle joint, you need to search for a cleft between the tibia and talus by flexion or extension of the ankle joint. Insert the needle just medial to the tibialis anterior tendon and direct it posterolaterally. The dose of methylprednisolone or triamcinolone to be administered is 20–40 mg.

Soft Tissue and Bursae Injections

Patients with trigger finger can be administered an injection of 15–20 mg methylprednisolone, mixed with 0.5 mL lidocaine. Insert the needle at an angle of 45°, just distal to the proximal palmar crease of the index finger, between the proximal and distal creases of the middle finger and distal to the distal palmar crease of the ring and little finger. The needle should be inserted in the distal direction.

An injection of 20–40 mg methylprednisolone, mixed with 1–2 mL of lignocaine, is administered for carpal tunnel syndrome, irrespective of the causes. Insert the needle 1 cm proximal to the distal palmar crease at the wrist and medial to the palmaris longus tendon (making it prominent by asking the patient to make a fist and, together with palmar flexion of the wrist joint, the palmaris longus tendon should become prominent. Insert the needle at an angle of 45° in the distal direction and a bit laterally (45°). In case the palmaris longus tendon cannot be located, insert the needle medial to the flexor digitorum superficialis or into the middle of the wrist.

In cases of de Quervain's tenosynovitis, you need to administer an injection of 15–20 mg methylprednisolone, with or without lignocaine. Insert the needle over the radial styloid process and pull it back a bit once it hits the bone. If there is no blood in the hub, you may administer the injection.

Ganglia over the dorsal aspect of the hand/wrist can be injected with up to 20 mg methylprednisolone. Insert the needle into the central part after aspirating the viscous translucent fluid.

For tennis elbow and golfer's elbow, give the patient an injection of 20 mg methyl-prednisolone. Ask him/her to indicate the point where the tenderness is the maximum and insert the needle until it touches the bone. Next, pull the needle back a millimeter and inject the drug in a fan-like fashion.

In pes anserine bursitis, the bursa can be injected with 20–40 mg methylprednisolone, mixed with 2–3 mL of lignocaine. Ask the patient to flex his/her knee at an angle of 90°. Look for the end point of the medial border of the semitendinosus tendon and mark the point. Extend the knee and insert the needle at an angle of 90°, until it touches the bone. Inject the drug in a fan-shape manner in an area with a diameter of 3 cm.

Plantar fasciitis requires an injection of 20–30 mg methylprednisolone, diluted with 1 mL of lignocaine. Insert the needle on the medial side, to a depth of 2 cm from the surface of the sole and toward the medial plantar tubercle of the calcaneus.

■ CONCLUSION

Intra-articular aspiration and injection constitute a simple and effective way of diagnosing and treating different joint conditions. In the hands of an expert, they are safe, easy to perform and often rewarding, provided that the differential diagnosis, various pathologies, and their applications are kept in mind.

■ ACKNOWLEDGMENT

Dr Jeet Patel

■ SUGGESTED READING

1. Courtney P, Doherty M. Joint aspiration and injection. Baillieres Best Pract Res Clin Rheumatol. 2005;19:345-69.
2. Habib GS, Saliba W, Nashashiki M. Local effects of intra-articular corticosteroids. Clin Rheumatol. 2010;29:347-56.
3. Koski JM. Ultrasound guided injections in rheumatology. J Rheumatol. 2000;27:2131-8.
4. Mace S, Vadas P, Pruzanski W. Anaphylactic shock induced by intraarticular injection of methylprednisolone acetate. J Rheumatol. 1997;24:1191-4.
5. Mader R, Lavi I, Luboshitzky R. Evaluation of the pituitary-adrenal axis function following single intraarticular injection of methylprednisolone. Arthritis Rheum. 2005; 52:924-8.
6. Pascual E, Doherty M. Aspiration of normal or asymptomatic pathological joints for diagnosis and research: Indications, technique and success rate. Ann Rheum Dis. 2009;68:3-7.
7. Schumacher HR Jr, Reginato AJ. Atlas of Synovial Fluid Analysis and Crystal Identification. Philadelphia: Lea and Febiger; 1991.

Liver Biopsy

Anil Arora

■ INTRODUCTION

Paul Ehrlich is credited with performing the first percutaneous liver biopsy in 1883 in Germany. A liver biopsy is usually the most specific test to assess the nature and severity of liver diseases. In addition, it can be useful in monitoring the efficacy of various treatments. There are several methods available for obtaining liver tissue: percutaneous biopsy, transjugular biopsy, laparoscopic biopsy, and fine-needle aspiration guided by ultrasonography or computed tomography. Each method has its advantages and disadvantages. The size of the biopsy specimen, which varies from 1 to 3 cm in length and 1.2 to 2 mm in diameter, represents $1/50,000$ of the total mass of the liver.

Usually, a specimen of a length of 1.5 cm is adequate for a diagnosis of diffuse liver disease. The number of portal triads present in the specimen is important. Most hepatopathologists are satisfied with a biopsy specimen containing at least 6–8 portal triads, especially in cases of chronic liver disease, in which the extent of injury may vary among portal triads.

■ INDICATIONS

- Diagnosis, grading and staging of alcoholic liver disease, nonalcoholic steatohepatitis (NASH), or autoimmune hepatitis
- Grading and staging of chronic hepatitis C or chronic hepatitis B
- Diagnosis of hemochromatosis in the index patient and his/her relatives, with quantitative estimation of iron levels
- Diagnosis of Wilson's disease, with quantitative estimation of copper levels
- Evaluation of cholestatic liver diseases, primary biliary cirrhosis, and primary sclerosing cholangitis
- Evaluation of abnormal results of biochemical tests of the liver in association with a serological workup that is negative or inconclusive
- Evaluation of the efficacy or adverse effects of treatment regimens (e.g., methotrexate therapy for psoriasis)
- Diagnosis of a liver mass
- Evaluation of the status of the liver after transplantation or of the donor liver before transplantation
- Evaluation of a fever of unknown origin, with a culture of tissue

■ COMPLICATIONS

Although the liver has a rich vascular supply, complications associated with percutaneous liver biopsy are rare. Sixty percent of complications occur within 2 hours and 96% within 24 hours of the procedure.

Approximately 1–3% of patients require hospitalization for complications after a liver biopsy, especially if the procedure was performed with a Tru-cut biopsy needle. Pain and hypotension are the predominant complications for which patients are hospitalized.

Minor complications after percutaneous liver biopsy include:
- Transient and localized discomfort at the site of the biopsy
- Pain that requires analgesia
- Mild and transient hypotension (due to a vasovagal reaction).

The rare complications include:
- Biliary ascites
- Bile pleuritis
- Bile peritonitis
- Pneumothorax
- Hemothorax
- Subcutaneous emphysema
- Pneumoperitoneum

■ CONTRAINDICATIONS

The absolute contraindications are:
- An uncooperative patient
- A history of unexplained bleeding
- Tendency to bleed
- Prothrombin time 3–5 seconds greater than in control
- Platelet count of <50,000/mm
- Unavailability of blood for transfusion
- Suspected hemangioma or other vascular tumor
- Inability to identify an appropriate site for biopsy by percussion or ultrasonography
- Suspicion of echinococcal cysts in the liver.

The relative contraindications are:
- Morbid obesity
- Ascites
- Hemophilia
- Infection in the right pleural cavity or below the right hemidiaphragm.

■ TRANSJUGULAR LIVER BIOPSY

After percutaneous puncture of the right internal jugular vein, introduce a catheter into the right hepatic vein with the help of fluoroscopy. Perform a needle biopsy of the liver through the catheter. According to various studies, the rate of complications associated with transjugular liver biopsy ranges from 1.3 to 20.2% and mortality ranges from 0.1 to 0.5%.

Indications

The indications for transjugular liver biopsy are:

- Severe coagulopathy
- Massive ascites
- Massive obesity
- Suspected vascular tumor or peliosis hepatis
- Need for ancillary vascular procedures (e.g., transjugular intrahepatic portosystemic shunting, and venography)
- Failure of percutaneous liver biopsy.

■ PITFALL OF LIVER BIOPSY—SAMPLING ERROR

Although liver biopsy clearly provides important diagnostic and prognostic information and helps define treatment plans, one must recognize that it may be associated with sampling variability. A smaller, but substantial proportion of biopsies were discordant by at least two stages. The interpretation of biopsies is subjective. Even among the pathologists involved in the development of the staging criteria, the interobserver and intraobserver concordance with respect to the fibrosis stage was 78 and 75%, respectively, but that with respect to inflammatory activity and fat burden was <50%.

■ ACKNOWLEDGMENT

Praveen Sharma

■ SUGGESTED READING

1. Bravo AA, Sheth SG, Chopra S. Liver biopsy. N Engl J Med. 2001;344:495-500.
2. Piccinino F, Sagnelli E, Pasquale G, Giusti G. Complications following percutaneous liver biopsy. A multicentre retrospective study on 68,276 biopsies. J Hepatol. 1986; 2:165-73.
3. Ratziu V, Charlotte F, Heurtier A, Gombert S, Giral P, Bruckert E, et al. Sampling variability of liver biopsy in nonalcoholic fatty liver disease. Gastroenterology. 2005; 128:1898-906.
4. Rockey DC, Caldwell SH, Goodman ZD, Nelson RC, Smith AD; American Association for the Study of Liver Diseases. Liver biopsy. Hepatology. 2009;49:1017-44.

Lumbar Puncture

Ish Anand

■ INTRODUCTION

Lumbar puncture is performed to obtain cerebrospinal fluid (CSF) from the spinal sub-arachnoid space for diagnostic or therapeutic purposes.

■ INDICATIONS

- The procedure is required for the diagnosis of meningitis, which may be viral, bacterial, fungal, tubercular, parasitic, carcinomatous, etc.
- It is performed for the diagnosis of subarachnoid hemorrhage (SAH) in patients in whom computed tomography (CT) or magnetic resonance imaging (MRI) of the brain does not show blood.
- The examination of CSF is helpful in the diagnosis of several disorders. Guillain–Barré syndrome may be diagnosed if albuminocytological dissociation is found. A finding of oligoclonal bands may be indicative of multiple sclerosis, JC virus may indicate progressive multifocal leukoencephalopathy and antimeasles antibodies may indicate subacute sclerosing panencephalitis (SSPE).
- A normal CSF examination and high CSF opening pressure are prerequisites for the diagnosis of idiopathic intracranial hypertension.
- In a patient suspected of having normal pressure hydrocephalus, the drainage of CSF is diagnostic. If the patient's symptoms are relieved by the procedure, the diagnosis is confirmed. Such patients are helped by CSF shunting surgery.

■ CONTRAINDICATIONS

These may be relative or absolute.

Absolute Contraindications

- A skin infection at the site of needle insertion is an absolute contraindication.
- Lumbar puncture should not be done if the intracranial pressure is raised, with unequal pressures in the supratentorial and infratentorial compartments. This can be assessed by CT or MRI of the brain which might show midline shift of brain, posterior fossa space-occupying lesions, and loss of suprachiasmatic cistern, basilar cisterns, superior cerebellar cistern, or quadrigeminal plate cistern. A lumbar puncture done in this condition may lead to coning and pressure over the brainstem, leading to catastrophic consequences.

Relative Contraindications

- Increased intracranial pressure
- Bleeding diathesis and the patient being on anticoagulants and antiplatelet agents
- Intracranial space-occupying lesions that do not fulfill the absolute contraindications criteria.

A CT scan of the brain should be performed before lumbar puncture if the patient:
- Is >60 years of age
- Is immunocompromised, has focal neurological deficits on examination, has papilledema, has had an epileptic attack in the preceding week, or has a history of intracranial lesions
- Is in altered sensorium.

◼ EQUIPMENT

A lumbar puncture tray should contain sterile dressing, sterile gloves, sterile drape, an antiseptic solution with skin swabs, lidocaine 1% without epinephrine, a 10-mL syringe with a needle, four plastic test tubes with caps (these should be numbered), lumbar puncture needles of 20 and 22 gauges, three-way stopcock, and manometer.

◼ TECHNIQUE

- Explain the procedure in great detail and obtain a signed informed consent
- Carry out an intradermal lignocaine sensitivity test 30 minutes before the procedure
- The patient must be in the lateral decubitus position, with the chin, hips, and knees flexed toward the chest. You my place a pillow between the legs. Alternatively, you may have the patient seated, with the neck flexed. The patient should lean forward, supported by the back of a chair. The sitting position is especially convenient in the case of obese patients because it makes confirming the midline easier **(Figs. 1 to 4)**.
- Palpate the right and left posterior superior iliac crests to locate the L3–L4 interspace. Move your fingers medially toward the spine. You may wear unsterile gloves during this process. Mark the entry site with a thumbnail or a marker **(Fig. 5)**.
- Wear sterile gloves and prepare the equipment. Open the numbered plastic tubes and place them upright. Assemble the stopcock on the manometer. Draw the lidocaine into the 10-mL syringe.
- Clean the skin with skin swabs and antiseptic solution, starting at the selected interspace and moving outward in a circular motion to include at least one interspace above and below.
- Place a sterile drape below the patient and a fenestrated drape on the patient. Use the 10-mL syringe to administer lignocaine **(Fig. 6)**.
- Wait for a few minutes. Then stabilize the 20- or 22-gauge needle with the index finger and thumb and advance it through the skin with a mild push. You should push the bevel of the needle in such a way that it does not cut the longitudinal dural fibers. It should face upward in the lateral recumbent position and toward the right or left in the sitting position.

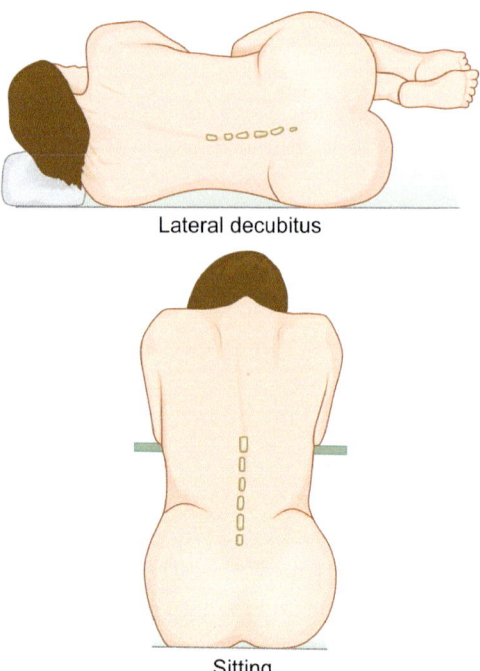

Lateral decubitus

Sitting

Fig. 1: Correct position for lumbar puncture.

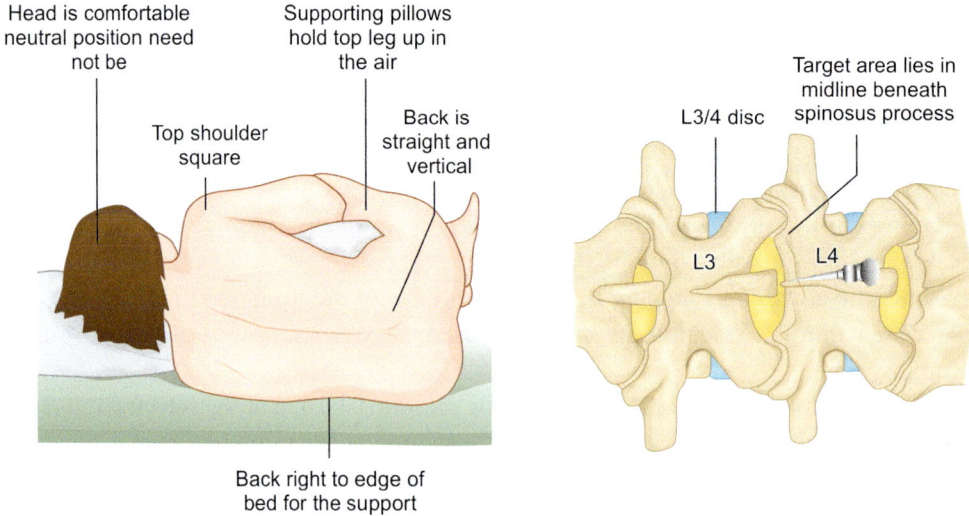

Head is comfortable neutral position need not be

Top shoulder square

Supporting pillows hold top leg up in the air

Back is straight and vertical

L3/4 disc

Target area lies in midline beneath spinosus process

L3

L4

Back right to edge of bed for the support

Fig. 2: Correct position (Cont.).

- Insert the needle at a slightly cephalad angle, directing it toward the umbilicus and push slowly. Remove the stylet after 4–5 cm of the needle has gone into check for CSF flow through the needle. If there is no fluid, insert the stylet into the needle and repeat the procedure.

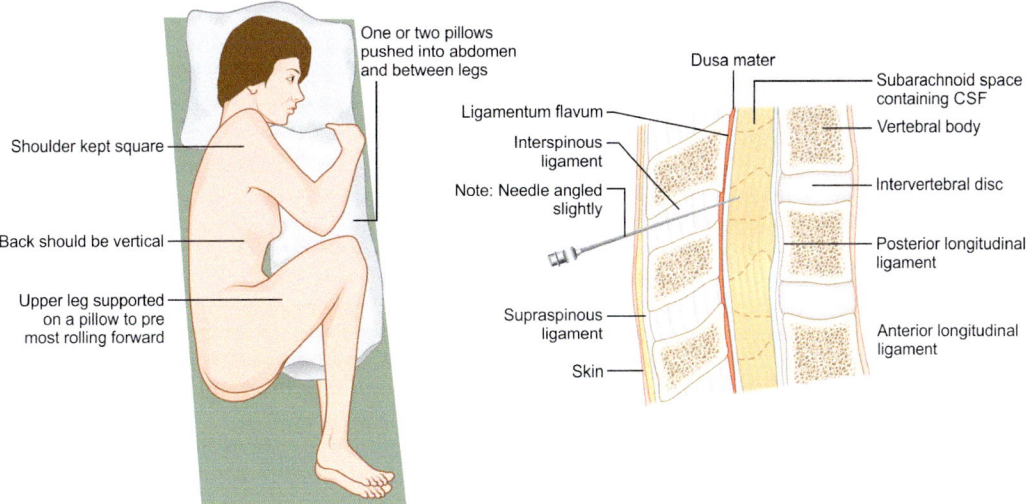

Fig. 3: Correct position seen from above with needle correctly inserted.

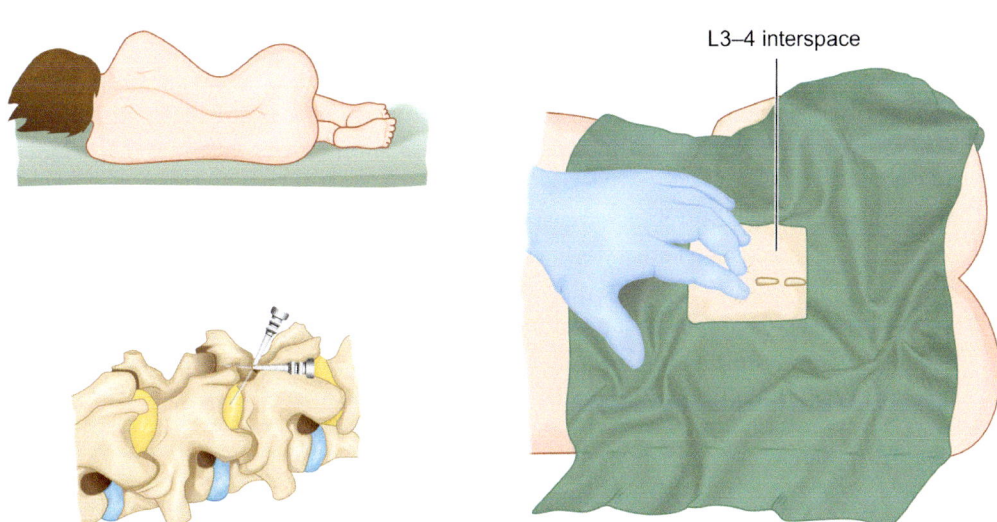

Fig. 4: Incorrect position for lumbar puncture (Rokeby venus position).

Fig. 5: Exposure of L3-L4 interface.

Introduce the needle a few millimeters at a time. Most of the time, small movements of the needle, either advancing it or removing it, helps to get a successful tap.
- The opening pressure of the CSF is measured in the lateral recumbent position. Even if the procedure is done in the sitting position, the patient must be shifted to the lateral recombinant position. The legs of the patient must be straight. When fluid starts flowing through the needle, attach the manometer to it through the stopcock and measure the height of the fluid column.

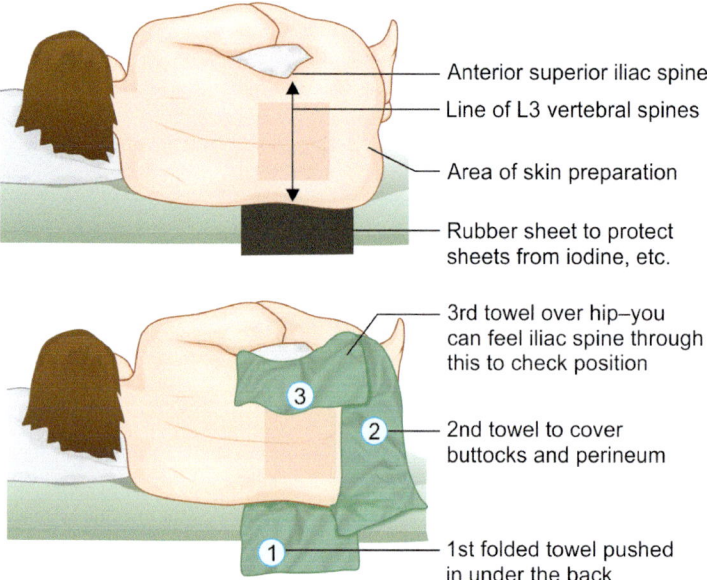

Anterior superior iliac spines

Line of L3 vertebral spines

Area of skin preparation

Rubber sheet to protect
sheets from iodine, etc.

3rd towel over hip—you
can feel iliac spine through
this to check position

2nd towel to cover
buttocks and perineum

1st folded towel pushed
in under the back

Fig. 6: Draping for the procedure.

- Collect approximately 1.5–2 mL of CSF in the four test tubes. Calculate the amount of fluid required before starting the procedure as it is an invasive procedure that cannot be repeated.
- After collecting the CSF, replace the stylet and remove the needle. Clean the skin at the puncture site and cover it with a sterile dressing. The patient should be placed in the supine position.
- Send the collected sample for laboratory tests, including cell count and differential count, glucose and protein levels, Gram stain, fungal stain, AFB stain, bacterial culture and sensitivity, and other tests indicated by clinical diagnosis.

■ COMPLICATIONS

Most of the time, the procedure is well tolerated by the patient, and there are no complications. In case there is a dry tap or bloody tap, repeat the procedure after a gap of 1 or 2 days. Infection, hemorrhage, and postpuncture brain herniation are rare complications and are unlikely to occur if asepsis is maintained and all the contraindications are considered before doing the procedure.

A headache is a common complication of lumbar puncture. It is more common in younger patients, and is mostly seen a day after the procedure. The probable etiology is the continued leakage of CSF from the puncture site. The headache is present on sitting and standing and is relieved when lying down. In some cases, the headache is severe and may be associated with vomiting. It may be relieved by increasing the oral intake of fluids, resting in bed, and analgesic medicines. It usually does not last for >5–7 days.

Dysesthesia is an uncommon complication and usually occurs in the legs due to the irritation of nerve roots by the spinal needle. This complication too settles with time, but in some cases, gabapentin or pregabalin may be need to be prescribed for a short time.

◼ SUGGESTED READING

1. Medscape. (2020). Lumbar Puncture Technique. [online]. Available from: https://emedicine. medscape.com/article/80773-technique#c5 [Last accessed September, 2022].

42

Urinary Catheterization: How to do it Safely?

Ajay Sharma

■ INTRODUCTION

Urinary catheterization is a procedure in which a tube, mostly a Foley catheter, is inserted into the bladder through the urethra. It is performed for a variety of indications and its purpose is drainage of the bladder. While the procedure is simple and straightforward in the absence of urethral pathology, it can be traumatic and inappropriate, and can give rise to complications and morbidity. Almost all the problems associated with it can be avoided by paying attention to a few basic details.

When considering catheterization, you need to keep the following in mind:

- *The age of the patient*: This will give you an idea of the size of the urethra, which is important for deciding on the size of the catheter.
- *Gender*: Female patients can tolerate catheters of a larger size than male patients.
- *Reason for inserting the catheter*: You must assess whether the patient is likely to need long-term or short-term catheterization because this will determine the type of catheter (latex or silicon) to be used.
- *Previous history of difficulty in passing urine*: Knowing the history will help in anticipating any difficulty in catheterization.

■ ARMAMENTARIUM

You should keep the following items ready: A catheter of the desired size, xylocaine jelly, gloves, a syringe with 10 mL saline or water, Betadine, and small drapes. Make sure that the patient has complete privacy. Ask the attendants, if any, to leave. Explain the procedure to the patient and reassure him/her that it will not hurt much.

■ RULES/GUIDELINES FOR CHOOSING CATHETER

Smaller is better. The presence of a catheter is injurious for the urethra as it can cause traumatic (frictional) ulcers, as well as an increase in urethral secretions, which can get infected. Catheters also cause meatal ulceration, leading to meatal or submeatal stenosis. To minimize this problem, the catheter should not fit snugly to the urethral wall. Urethral secretions should have enough room to pass out.

In the case of short-term drainage, a 14-Fr catheter is optimum for adequate drainage. The usual latex catheter will do. You may use a 14-Fr catheter even for longer term drainage, but it often gets blocked by phosphate crystals. In such cases, 16 Fr is a good choice and a silicon catheter is a better option.

■ PROCEDURE

The technique for the procedure should ideally involve no touch, and should be aseptic and atraumatic. Further, it should be painless for the patient. The first step is to prepare the area by putting drapes around the penis (perineum in the case of a female). This is done to prevent the catheter from accidentally touching the skin. Then clean the area with Betadine (not spirit or Savlon).

Using the nozzle supplied in the pack, instill the xylocaine jelly, which serves both as an anesthetic and a lubricant. In the case of males, instill the whole tube (30 mL). Do it gradually, without distending the urethra acutely. In the case of females, 5–10 mL will suffice. The general rule is to instill the jelly generously.

Wait for 3–5 minutes after instilling the jelly and then insert the catheter, slightly stretching the penis and holding it in a vertical position. In females, you need to separate the labia majora so that the catheter does not touch the surrounding area. Sometimes, it is difficult to locate the meatus in female patients. You should be sure of its location before attempting catheterization.

While inserting the catheter, you should pay attention to the tactile sensation you experience. A feeling of slight resistance is necessary in order to be gentle. In a male patient, insert the catheter almost completely up to the beginning of the balloon channel (bifurcation). This ensures that the balloon is placed well inside the bladder and not in the urethra. Once you are certain of this, fill the balloon with not more than 10 mL of sterile water/saline. A larger quantity of water would cause irritation to the bladder and spasms. If the catheter is not inserted fully, it might get inflated in the urethra. This would cause severe rupture of the urethra, leading to bleeding and consequently a urethral stricture.

When you are not sure whether the catheter has entered the bladder fully, first aspirate the urine and if all is well, fill the balloon. Do not rely on the passage of urine through the catheter as an indicator of its position, as the eye of the catheter is proximal to the balloon, which can still be inflated in the urethra. Briefly put, be very careful not to inflate the catheter in the urethra. This problem rarely occurs among females as the urethra is short.

Once you have inflated the balloon, pull the catheter out till the neck of the bladder and secure it to the abdomen or thigh. This should be done very lightly and it is important to make sure that the patient is comfortable. Clean the parts well. Avoid occlusive dressings.

In a male patient, do not forget to pull the prepuce forward. If you fail to do so, he will develop paraphimosis.

The following are some difficult situations and ways of handling them:

- *Penile edema*: This leads to extreme swelling of the prepuce so much so that the meatus is not visible. Gently squeeze the penis and prepuce to displace the water. This method works most of the time.
- *Phimosis*: In this condition, the prepuce cannot be pulled back over the tip of the penis. This causes the prepuce to become swollen and stuck, which may slow down or stop the flow of blood to the tip of the penis. Gently dilate the preputial opening, just enough to

allow catheterization. Sometimes, you may need to make a dorsal slit after administering local anesthesia.

- *Meatal stenosis and balanitis xerotica obliterans*: These require dilatation following penile block.
- *Urethral stricture*: This refers to a narrowing of the urethra that restricts the flow of urine from the bladder. It should be dealt with by an expert, who may have to carry out dilatation. If the stricture is too tight and if an endoscopic procedure is not possible, suprapubic catheterization should be performed.
- *Female hypospadias*: In female hypospadias, the meatus which is located just at the vaginal opening or slightly on the anterior vaginal wall. Locate it by gently putting a finger into the vagina and then pull out the meatus.

Children pose different problems due to not cooperating. Choose the appropriate size, from 5–6 Fr feeding tube to 10 Fr Foley catheter, using the same principles.

Catheter care: Care of the catheter may be taken either by a nurse or the patient Encourage daily washing with water and soap.

■ CONCLUSION

Though this procedure is simple, one should not be casual about it. Initially, you should do it under supervision. Do not hesitate to call a senior in case of difficulty, else you may cause harm to the patient due to your lack of expertise, which will develop with time.

Index